COMMON SPORTS INJURIES BETWEEN TEAM & INDIVIDUAL SPORTS COMPETITION

By PAVIN

ABSTRACT

1   Athletic Injuries

Injuries in sports due to acute distress or repetitive pressure related to athletic activities. Games wounds will affect bones or delicate tissue (tendons, muscles, ligaments). Consistently, a great deal of people (everything being equal) inside the world partake in physical activity and games exercises, from affiliation football field to softball jewels and Kabaddi courts. It's called playing at the same time, however wears exercises are more than play. Cooperation in sports enhances physical wellness, coordination and self-restraint, and give kids and individual profitable chances to learn collaboration. Amusement and games can likewise bring about wounds some minor, some genuine, and still others bringing about long lasting medicinal issues. **(Ajmer Singh, 2012)**

Sports carry an element of risk in the form of injury. In fact, there is no sport-whether amateur or professional-where injury does not occur. In some sports, chance injury may be much more due to the nature of the sport itself; in others, it may be less. The athletic injury may be as simple and insignificant as a bruise on the knee or elbow and as serious and fatal as a thigh fracture or skull smash. Athletic injuries occur from two different mechanisms: macrotruma, and microtruma. **Macrotrauma**-a deeply distressing experience-is a sudden injury from a major force. This could for example, be due to a bad fall from a horizontal (or parallel) bar or a ball hit during play in field hockey or cricket. Such situations abound in almost all sports, and can cause fractures, sprains or ligament, muscle strains (tear) and bruises or contusion, which are commonly termed as acute injuries. **Microtrauma** is due to repetitive injury over a long period of time and these injuries are also termed overuse. Types of injuries include stress fracture, little league elbow and shoulder impingement syndrome. Most sports injuries involve muscoskeletal system.

1.1.1 The international Federation and Sports Medicine

The first important attempt should be to bring together physicians interested in physical exercise and related problems, and to define as area of interest in sports medicine. It appears to have been the establishment of a separate section of "Hygiene of Physical Exercise" by Dr. A. Malwitz at the World Hygiene Exposition in Dresden in 1911. In March 1913, a medical congress dealing with sports was held in Paris, it dealt chiefly with physical therapy and the physiology of exercise. World War I brought an end to such meetings for a period of 15 years.

In February 14, 1928 during the second winter Olympic games at Saint Moritz, Switzerland, Drs. W. Knoll of Switzerland and F. Laterjet of France called together 33 physicians who have attending the team of 11 nations. This meeting established a committee whose function was to plan for the First International Congress of Sports Medicine to take place during the games of the IX Olympic at Amsterdam in August of the same year and to propose and plan an organization for a permanent international assembly of sports medicine. Dr.Mallwitz, Secretary and other members was Drs. Dybowski of Poland and Latarjet and Buytendijk of Holland.

When the congress met in Amsterdam, 281 physicians and specialists in physical education representing 20 different countries were present. The first Constitution of the Association International Medico-Sportive (AIMS) was adopted and F.J.J. Buytenkijk of Holland was elected President. Three principle purposes were included in the first constitution:

1. To inaugurate scientific research in biology, psychology and sociology in relation to sports.
2. To encourage the study of medical complications encountered in physical exercise in sports in collaboration with the various international sports federations, and
3. To establish international congresses on the area of sports medicine to be held throughout and at the site of the quadrennial Olympic games.

Although a physician from New York City named Brown was chosen to organize a congress at the X-Olympiad in Los Angeles in 1932, the meeting was never held, probably because no organized activities in sports medicine existed in the United State at that time. It was consequently agreed to hold the second congress at Turin, Italy in September 1933. By this time Dr. Laterjet was serving as President, following the resignation of Dr. Buytendijk. The topics discussed were grouped under nine headings: anthropology, charts for evaluating physical fitness, the medical control of sports, the kidney and the sports, respiratory physiology, fatigue, and women in sports. It was established that a general assembly of the new association would be held every four years at the time of the International Congress and its name was changed to the Federation International Medico-Sportive et Scientifique (FIMS)

1.1.2 Future Perspective of Sports Medicine
Through the world sports medicine is recognized as a specialty of medical practice. It is not well established in every country as yet, which might be expected because interest has crystallized recently. In every place where sports medicine has become well established it maintains a close relationship to those agencies and individuals who are concerned with all aspects of the regulation of physical training, physical education, and sports. The establishment of centers for the medical control of sports has provided facilities and funds for research in sports medicine in which the persons engaged in these various disciplines may collaborate. Sports medicine has made and should continue to make important contributions to medical knowledge and practice. In therapy one must consider especially the contributions in therapeutic exercise or medical gymnastics that have come from the interest of physicians on sports and physical education. The earlier and more aggressive approach to the operative treatment of severe joint injuries is a direct outgrowth of experience derived from the care of athlete

At the same time, sports medicine has made contributions to physical education, among which is notably the development of adapted physical education. Through research in the physiology of exercise the way has been opened to improved performance in sports, especially in endurance events.

Finally, although great studies have occurred in the development of preventive medicine through sports medicine, in this area lays the greatest possibility for future achievements. Physical recreation will play an increasingly important part in the lives of the world's populations in the future. The steps taken so far by sports medicine to make it safe as well as enjoyable must be continued and greatly expanded. Although we believe that a lifetime of vigorous physical activity favors good health and longevity, the final and conclusive proof of this theory has yet to be made **(Pande, 1987)**

1.1.3 Sports Physiotherapy in India

Sports medicine in India is still in its infancy, so that sports physiotherapy as a part of the overall scope of sports medicine has not been very highly developed as yet, although it has already certainly made a significant contribution to the management of sports injuries. There are seven physiotherapy schools for basic training in India. Most of the courses last for two years, leading to a diploma or degree according to the school. Two schools, at Bombay and Baroda (Gujarat), have university-based courses lasting three years or slightly longer, leading to a degree. Sports medicine is included in the basic curriculum. However, there is no really specialized training in sports physiotherapy in Indian as yet, and there are very few jobs available within sports clubs or the sports federations. The board of control for cricket is one of the few bodies to employ physiotherapists. There for working at a sports center like the National Institute of Sports provide rare experience for Indian physiotherapists. The National Institute of Sports in Patiala is also the headquarter of the Indian Association of Sports Medicine (IASM). From time to time short courses are held there for doctors and physiotherapists who are mainly in general practice and who require orientation in the management of sports injuries. These courses are conducted by Indian expert in collaboration with visiting foreign experts, mainly from the Soviet Union an East and West Germany. In 1979, 26 doctors from 11 Asian countries attended the first three-week course in sports medicine at the National Institute of Sports in Patiala held under the aegis of the Federation International de Medicine Sportive (FIMS) and the International Olympic Committee (IOC), and leading to the Asian Diploma in Sports Medicine. In 1983, a three-week sports physiotherapy course conducted by the East German Expert Professor (Mrs) Helga Schmidt was attended by 31 physiotherapists and doctors. Since 1987, the National Institute of Sports has been running its own one-year diploma course in sports medicine. **(Grinsogono, 1989)**

2   Research Procedure and Methodology

Injuries caused by participation in various games for sports are more common today since more people are involved in sports of all type. Many new and often high risk sports now exist, for example, hand gliding. The age range of competitors has widened with, children started sports, younger and adults continuing longer. Professional athlete need to be fitter today than those athletes in previous year. They compete more frequently and often at a higher level, as witnessed by the speed with which records fall.

In India, the sports, still is an upcoming field. Now a day the athletes are going towards professionalism. With this cause the standard of sports is also increasing and the level, nature and type of injuries among the Indian male athletes are increasing. So it is very important for the professional of physical education and sports to know the different kind of injuries among Indian male and female athletes. But the present study focuses on male athletes only.

The purpose of the study was to compare the common sports injuries in team and individual sports competition. An attempt had been made by the researcher to endure the dimensions of the injuries in team and individual sports competition by identifying the different aspects related to sports injuries.

This chapter describes the procedure adopted for selection of subjects (source of data), selection of variables, development of inventory, and administration of inventory, collection of data and statistical analysis of data.

2.1 Selection of the Subjects

As per the advises of the experts including my supervisor and prevailing practices, keeping in view the feasibility and purpose of the study, it was resolve to collect data from following sources.

- Sportspersons (Male only)
- Team Game
- Individual Game

Keeping in view the statistical guidelines and feasibility in mind the numbers of samples from each category were planned as per the advice of the statisticians. The detail descriptions of sources are explained in table: 3.1.

Table 2-1 : Classification of Sample

GAME TYPE	SPORTS	SAMPLE (N)
	Cricket	25
	Baseball	25
	Kabaddi	25
	Basketball	25
Team Games	Hockey	25
	Football	25
	Total Subjects from Team Game	**150**
	Wrestling	25
	Weight Lifting	25
	Badminton	25

	Boxing	25
Individual	Gymnastic	25
Games	Judo	25
	Total Subjects from Individual game	**150**
	Grand Total (150+150)	**300**

From the population a total 300 samples were selected through random sampling technique from Team and Individual sports competition, out of the total sample half of the sample (N=150) were from team game and (N=150) were from individual game. Six games were selected for team game and Six games were selected for individual game (see table 3.1). 25 male sportsperson of national/inter-university/international from each delimited games were planned for sampling. The age of selected samples were ranged from 17 to 35 years.

2.2   Selection of Variables

The research scholar critically studies the available scientific literature from sport medicine books, journals, magazines and periodicals etc. related to sports injuries. As well as keeping in view the feasibility criteria, availability of the instruments, experts' opinion and the purpose of the present study following variables have been selected:

Under the objective of type, classification and distribution of common sports injuries following variables have been selected:

1. Common sports injuries
2. Body parts associated with sports injuries.
3. Time lost in days due to injury.
4. Injury occurred during match and training.
5. New and Recurrent injuries.
6. Injury type (soft, bone, and joint injuries)

7. playfields and injuries

Under the objective of sports injuries severity following variables have been selected:

1. Injury associated with the greatest time loss in team games.
2. Injury associated with the greatest time loss in individual games.
3. Injury associated with the greatest time loss in each selected game.

Under the objective of reasons of sports injuries following variables have been selected:

1. Intrinsic reasons of injuries
2. Extrinsic reasons of injuries

2.3 Development of Injury Report Inventory

The distinction and interpretation of sports injury statistics are relevant to role of athletic trainers, who are responsible, in part, for promoting the safety of sports in society. It is therefore important for athletic trainers in all setting to gain an understanding of the cause of and risk factors for sports related injury. To do this athlete's trainers must be able to accurately measure and assess injury related data. So, the development of injury inventory is a most important factor in sports injury research.

In order to gain knowledge about athletic injuries, it is necessary to record and report injuries. It is essential that those who report injuries be properly educated about the terms and definitions of injury, what information to gather, and how to record this information on the appropriate forms. There must be completeness, uniformity, accuracy, and standardization of methodology to be able to make meaningful comparisons among different reports of injuries.

A data collection system must consider exactly what information is to be gathered and who will record the data. The forms utilized must be appropriate for the task. All reporters should be carefully educated, clearly understanding and all terms and definitions. Completeness, accuracy, and uniformity are essential in conducting any injury study.

STEP-I   Objectives of the Sports Injury Inventory

1. To study the demographic information of selected sample.
2. Percentage distribution, frequency distribution, percentage ranking of injuries in selected games.
3. Incidence rate, percentage distribution, frequency distribution and percentage ranking of body part associated of injuries in selected games.
4. Distribution of injury severity in relation to days lost from training and competition due to injury in selected games.
5. Assessment of match or training injuries.
6. Assessment of new and recurrent injuries.
7. To assess the type of injury (soft/bone/joint)
8. To assess the playfield and injury relationship.
9. To find out the possible reasons of injury (intrinsic and extrinsic)
10. Comparison of sports injuries between team and individual games.

STEP-II   Selection of Item

1. Demographic information includes Name, Age, Height, Weight, Game, Playing Position, Gender, Region, Level of Competition, Playing Experience, Training Hours and University.
2. List down the injuries you have experienced due to your games/sports.
3. Body part associated with injuries.
4. Time lost in days (for obtained severity).
5. When Injury occurred? In Match or Training

6. Injury classification. (New and Recurrent Injuries)
7. Injury Type. (soft tissue, bone and joint injuries)
8. Type of playfield related to injury.
9. Possible causes of injury which are listed.

STEP-III   Development of Blue Print

Then the blue print was prepared comprising the above inventory, there after subjected for trail run.

STEP-IV   Trial Run

After the trial run few modifications were made based on the most commonly agreed language, inventory, questioning etc.

STEP-V   Reliability, Validity and Objectivity of the Inventory.

The developed inventory was obtained open ended responses. So, the inventory was considered sufficiently reliable and objective as it was designed under the guidance of number of experts by adopting phase wise trial run and followed by required improvement based on most commonly agreed language, presentation, nature of inventory, nature of questioning and required/responses to design the final shape of the inventory ultimately. Thus, keeping in view the feasibility, the statistical means of reliability were also established. As earlier said that the inventory consisted of open-ended responses so, following method of reliability were used:

Inter-Rater Reliability

In statistics, inter-rater reliability, inter-rater agreement, or concordance, is the degree of agreement among raters. It gives a score of how much consistency, or consent, there is in the ratings given by adjudicators, and it is one of the aspects of test validity. It is useful in refining the tools given to human judges, for example by determining if a particular scale is appropriate for determining a particular variable. If various raters do not agree, either the scale is defective or the raters need to be re-trained. There are a number of statistics which can be used to determine inter-rater reliability. Different statistics are appropriate for different types of measurement. Some options are: **joint-probability of agreement, Cohen's kappa, Scott's pi** and the related **Fleiss' kappa, inter-rater correlation, concordance correlation coefficient** and **intra-class correlation**. For established the reliability of present sports injury inventory Intera-class correlation method was used.

Intra-Class Correlation Coefficient

There are several types of this method and one of them defined as, "the proportion of variance of an observation due to between-subject variability in the true scores". he range of the intra-class correlation may be between 0.0 and 1.0. The intra-class correlation will be high when there is little variation between the scores given to each item by the raters, e.g. if all raters give the same, or similar scores to each of the items. The obtained value of Intra-class correlation was .880 which show that inventory was significant reliable.

For detail regarding developed inventory please refer appendix

2.4   Administration of Injury Report Inventory

1. For each category of sample, by and large the research scholar has approached to them individually.
2. After ensuring the availability of time, the purpose of the study has been explained to the respondents.
3. Once they understood and agreed to responses and participated in the study, consent has been taken.
4. Thereafter required inventory has been distributed to the subjects and requested to read once carefully without giving any response.
5. Doubt or confusion of respondents were finally cleared or explained.

6. In case of language, the research scholar read out and explained the meaning of questions, and noted down the required response.

7. After ensuring that they have understood and concerned individual was prepared for responding, the required inventory was got filled up by the respondents.

2.5 Data Collection

The researcher personally visited the desired destinations to fulfillment their research work of sports injuries. The data has been collected from the All India Universities Competitions held at different campuses of Indian Universities. Each injury episode during training or match-play was outlined in a detailed injury report form that was completed by experts of sports medicines. The injury reports form comprise a questionnaire of the injury specific including, injury, body part associated, time lost due to injury (for severity purpose), injury classification, injury type, playing surface and reason of injury with match-play events associated with injuries. All injuries assessed after the confirmation of a physiotherapist whom were presented at the time of competition to ensure the accuracy of details when completing injury record documentation.

The description of the All India-University competitions where the data had been collected given below:

Table 2-2 Description of Events

Game	Date	Venue
Cricket	22-30 Nov 2017	M D U, Rohtak
Baseball	14-18 Nov 2017	M D U Rohtak
Kabaddi	19-23 Nov 2017	M. D. U, Rohtak
Basketball	26-30 Dec 2017	JMI. N. Delhi
Hockey	1st Oct 2017	NHIS, Delhi

Football	22-30 Nov 2017	D.B. University
Wrestling	3-5 Nov 2017	M D U, Rohtak
Wt. Lifting	4-6 Nov 2017	Chandigarh University, Mohali
Badminton	1-4 Dec 2017	M D U, Rohtak
Boxing	1-4 Feb 2018	Chandigarh
Gymnastic	15-18 Jan	KUK, Kurukshetra
Judo	22-24 Feb 2018	Chandigarh

2.6 Statistical Techniques Used for Analysis of the Data

The purpose of the present study was to compare the common sports injuries between team and individual sports competitions. For accomplish the study following statistical tools were used to analysis the raw data:

- Percentage
- Injury ranking
- Normal Curve Distribution
- Chi-square

Percentage

In its simplest form, percent mean per hundred. To definite a number between zero and one, percentage formula is used. It is defines as a number represented as a fraction of 100. Symbolized by the symbol = %, it is majorly used to compare and finding out ratios. The Percentage Formula is given as,

Percentage=————

Normal Curve Distribution

First step:

- Mean: —

- Standard Deviation: $\sqrt{\rule{0.8em}{0pt}}$

Second step

- A normal curve covers ±3σ
- : Total distance = 6σ
- To grade the injury severity into 5 categories in the normal curve within 6σ limit.
- Each grade curve = — = 1.2σ

Third Step:

Thus to find out the area covered by each grade in the normal curve i.e. ±3σ. Standard score formula $\{z = \rule{1.5em}{0pt}\}$ is employed to find out the range of each point to categorize the grade.

- Critical: x=3×SD+Mean
- Severe: x= 1.8×SD+Mean
- Serious: x=6×SD+Mean
- Moderate: x= -.6×SD+Mean
- Minor : x=-1.8×SD+Mean

Thus to calculate the lowest range, we have to calculate the lower limit here,

- X= -3×SD+Mean

Fourth step:

To get the range of all desired grade the upper limit of corresponding scale will be subtracted from the upper limit of next below.

Non Parametric Statistics

Non-parametric statistics makes weaker and fewer assumptions about the characteristic of the population distribution. Depend only sparingly on the latter, do not involve the population parameters, and can be applied irrespectively or sample size and population distribution or even for nomination or ordinal variables.

Where use:

- Non-parametric statistics can be applied to the data involving nominal or ordinal variables and too small sample or samples drawn from non-normally distributed population.
- Most non-parametric test that used for testing experimental hypothesis and for analyzing the observed frequencies and variance, are less complicated and speedier in calculation than parametric ones.
- Non-parametric tests are less appropriate than parametric tests for ratio and interval variables.
- Less powerful than that of parametric statistics.

Chi-square (x^2)

a non-parametric test is conventionally called the chi square test because the statistics computed for it has a x^2 sampling distribution. It is a generalized expression between a theoretical and actual distribution, i.e. an actual response as related to an expected responses. It can be used with either parametric or non-parametric data.

$$X^2 = \frac{(O \qquad i)}{}$$

Where,

O_i = frequency of occurrence or observed.

E_i = frequency of occurrence as indicated by some hypothesis or expected.

Chi-square Test of Independence.

x^2 test are used to find whether there is a significant association between two variables in a sample or the two variables are independent or each other.

3   FINDINGS

3.1   Findings in Distribution of Injuries in Team and Individual Games

Team Games: A total 532 frequencies of injuries were recorded during data collection in team games. Highest, (83) responses are of Abrasion which constitute 15.6% of the total responses. Injury rate (IR) of 'Abrasion' in Team games was 55.7% per 100 athletes. It means if there were 100 injuries occurred in team games then 56 (approximately) should be Abrasion. Second highest, (67) responses are of 'Sprain' which constitute 12.6% of the total responses and Injury rate was 45% respectively. Contusion, Muscle pull, Fracture and Ligament Rupture has also a considerable frequencies and their injury rate illustrate probability of their occurrence. Fracture and Ligament Rupture are severe injuries which may lead serious consequences in the career of a sportsperson. Some Meniscus Tear (1.1%) and Concussion (0.8%) were also observed which are also under the severe category.

Individual Games: A total 364 responses were retraced in Individual Games. Highest, 50 responses were Muscle Pull which constitutes 13.7% of the total responses. Injury rate of muscle pull was 34%, which shows a considerable amount of probability of occurrence in individual games. Second, highest (45) responses were contusion which constitute12.4% of the total sample and out of 100 injuries, the probability of Contusion is 31 approximately. 25 responses were Dislocation which shows a significant amount of injured respondents whose body parts were dislocated in individual games.

Game Wise: Muscle Pull and Abrasions found the highest probable injury in Cricket and Baseball. Sprain is one of the highest frequent injuries in Kabaddi, whereas Fracture and Sprain is frequent injuries in Basketball. Abrasion and Contusion in Hockey, Abrasion, Sprain and Contusion in Football, Fracture and Contusion and Wrestling, Strain and Blisters in Weight Lifting, Muscle Cramp, Muscle Pull and Sprain in Badminton, direct hit on Knuckles (Contusion) in Boxing, Fracture and Abrasion in Gymnastic, Dislocation and Abrasion in Judo is highest frequent injuries retraced during data collection.

3.2   Findings in Body Parts Associated with Injuries

Team Games: Knee is highest frequent body part associated with injuries in team games. A total 415 frequencies of body parts recorded during data collection. 56 responses are Knee which constitutes 13.5% of the total sample and probability of injury occurrence in knee is 48.3% respectively. Second highest responses are come from Ankle. 52 responses are Ankle which constitutes 12.5% of the total responses and probability is 44.8%. Whereas, Elbow, Shoulder, Thigh, Calf, Eyebrow, Hamstring Muscle, Hand, Fingers has also considerable amount of responses noticed.

Individual Games: Knee is found highest body parts associated with injuries Individual Game also. A total 438 responses were noticed. 56 responses are Knee which constitutes 12.8% of the total sample, second, highest body part is Shoulder. 38 responses are Shoulder and which covers 8.7% of the total responses and probability of injury occurrence of shoulder is 27.5% out of hundred times. It is observed that Lumber Vertebrae which is a vital body part has 32 responses which make 7.3% of the total response and probability is 23.2% is a significant amount. Elbow, Fingers, Thigh, Palm, Face, Hamstring Muscle, Wrist, Thumb, Calf, Shin are also found significant association with injuries.

Game Wise: In Cricket Elbow, Lumber Vertebrae and Shoulder have the highest association with injuries. Shoulder is also associated in Baseball also. Knee, elbow, chin and ankle are highly probable to injury in Kabaddi. Ankle and Knee in Basketball, Knee, elbow and hamstring muscle in Hockey, Knee, ankle, thigh, calf, foot in Football, Knee in Wrestling, Lumber Vertebrae in Weight Lifting, Knee, ankle and shoulder in Badminton. Knuckles, nose, thumb and shoulder in Boxing. Shoulder and hand in Gymnastic. Knee, face, ankle and shoulder in Judo found to be most probable body parts associated with injuries. It is observed that mostly responses are come from knee in both team and individual games. It means knee has the highest probability to be injured in both type of games.

3.3 Findings in Injury Severity

In previous tables we interpreted only frequency of injury occurrence and most frequent body part associated with injuries. This section brings some important aspect of the present study. There are a huge difference between frequency of injury and severity of an injury. For instance, Abrasion is highest frequent injury in Team and Individual Games but as per the table it has last no. in the table. Severity shows the seriousness of the injury and it was based on the total days lost from practice and competition. It was assumed that an injured person would rest according to their injury severity. More rest mean more serious injury. It was observed that Meniscus Tear is a highest severe injury in Team Games with mean of 150 days lost from competition and practice. Second highest severe is Ligament Rupture within the mean of 129 days approximately. Whereas, the minimum and maximum values of resting days of Ligament rupture are 15±365 days which include partial tear to complete rupture. Next severe injury is fracture. The mean score of fracture is 63.61 days and minimum and maximum rest is 4±180 days which include stress to complicated fractures. Concussion and Low Back Pain are also found significant injuries in team games. In individual Games: Meniscus Tear is also considered severe injury in individual games. But there is a slightly difference in there score of the mean score of meniscus in individual games is 227.50 days (228 approximately). Some meniscus injuries were operated by doctors but after one year of rest and rehabilitation period the pain start again in knee. Mostly of cases told that operation of meniscus tear was not successful. Mean of Dislocation is 83 days in individual games and 34.53 days in team games because in team some subluxate (partial dislocate) were observed but due to the nature of the game complete dislocation were observed in Individual games. The mean score of Fracture is 78.43 which is also higher than the Fracture in Team games. For deep interpretation see table 4-42 in Chatper-4.

After analysis the results it was retraced that frequency of injuries is high in team games but severity of injuries are higher in individual games. Severity are classified on five rating scale on the basis of days lost from competition and practice. With the help of normal curve the score of Injury severity is distributed on three point rating scale (Minor, Moderate, and Severe,) to classified injury severity scale.

Figure 3-1 Normal Curve Drawn to Develop Three Point Scale for Injury Severity

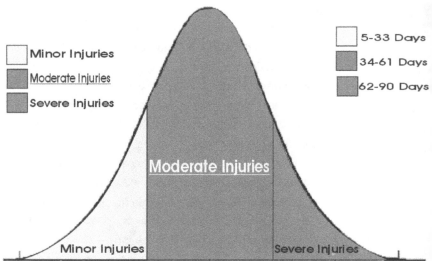

Table 3-1 Result for Injury Severity

Days	Severity
5-33	Minor Injuries
34-61	Moderate Injuries
62-90	Severe Injuries

The table 5.1 evident the grading of injury severity on five point rating scale. After injury occurred, if an injured individual will rest 5 to 33 days, his injury will be considered as minor injury. If he rest for 62 to 90 days, his injury will be considered as critical injury.

3.4 Findings in Match or Training Injuries

In **team games** a total 458 injuries were recorded. 260 injuries were occurred during match or competition which makes 56.76% of the total responses, whereas 198 injuries were occurred during training period which covered 43.24% of the total response. In **individual games** a total 262 injuries were noticed. 87 injuries were from match which constitute 33.20% of the total responses and 175 injuries were recorded from training which constitute 66.79% of the total sample. So, we can say that in team games the probability of injury occurrence is higher during match in comparison of training on the other hand occurrence of injuries is higher during training in Individual games.

As per **game wise** distribution of injuries, it was observed that Football has the higher rate of injury percentage in both match and training in team games. In individual sports Judo has higher injury prone sports.

3.5 Findings in New and Recurrent Injuries

A 'New injury' is defined as an injury which occur first time and 'Recurrent Injury' means, when same injury happens again. The percentage (51.01) of recurrent injuries is higher in team games and percentage distribution of new injuries is higher in individual games. Higher percentage of recurrent injuries shows the injury pattern of team games which show that a same injury is repeating again and again. It could be due to careless and other factors which should be considered in team games. Football and Judo from team and individual games has higher percentage of new and recurrent injuries also.

3.6 Findings in Soft Tissue, Bone and Joint Injuries

Football has higher rate of percentage of soft tissue and Joint injuries whereas, Basketball has the highest percentage of bone injuries in team games. In individual games 61 responses of soft tissue injuries were came from Judo which constitutes highest 35.46% of the total responses. 41 responses of frequencies of bone injuries were came from Boxing which covers highest 57.74% of the total responses. In Joint injuries Judo has also highest frequencies (22) which make 36.66% of the total responses. It is recommended that mostly of the injuries could be prevented if an individual use protective equipment's.

3.7 Findings in Surface Related Injuries

It was observed that in **team games** clay and natural grass field are highly prone to injuries. A significant amount of injuries were occurred on both surfaces. It was analyzed that wooden surface has the lowest amount of injuries percentage. So, it could be said that playing surface plays a significant role in injury prevention. In individual game highest injury prone surface was Mat. 107 responses of injuries were came from Mat which makes 59.77% of the total responses.

3.8 Findings in Injury Reasons

Intrinsic Reason: The reason of injuries was different in various team and individual sports. Improper warming-up is a cause of injury that occurred highest and common in all the sports. Different cause of Injuries in sports varying from one sports to another and affected by various factors. Twisting is a reason of injury that was highest in individual games. It was also an interesting fact that majority of the sportsperson did not know the exact reason of injury that's why they select an option 'Unknown' given in injury report form.

Extrinsic Reason: The various extrinsic reasons were observed in different team and individual sports. Field/playground is a reason of injury that occurred highest in **team games**. This is a very important and considerable reason which can be prevented. At college level sports we have not sufficient and latest facilities for instance, wooden surfaces, artificial grass, AstroTurf etc. The lack of these facilities may lead to injuries in sports. Fall or slip is a second reason that is highest in team games. Careless as a injury reason has also observed considerable responses. It is the part of sports person. When an individual is careless during practice or match then coach duty is to identify the exact reason of their carelessness. In **individual games** collision/impact is a reason of injury that is highest percentage distribution. Second highest extrinsic reason of injury is fall or slip which can be occurred due to various causes such as balance, proper footwear, proper technique, collision etc. it is also observed in extrinsic reasons that some sportsperson did not know the exact reason of injury. That's why a considerable amount of recurrent injuries were noticed in team and individual sports. The knowledge of sports medicine and injury pattern should be essential part of the training of a sports person.

3.9 Findings in comparison of sports injuries.

To compare the ordinal data of sports injuries between team and individual sports non-parametric statistics (chi-square) was used.

Table 3-2 Association between Injuries and Game Type

Sr.No.	(Injuries)	(df)	(χ^2)	Asymp.sig.
1	Abrasion	1	**31.539**	**.000**
2	Blisters	1	.655	.418
3	Contusion	1	1.109	.292
4	Incision	1	8.518	.004
5	Laceration	1	9.015	.003
6	Dislocation	1	2.448	.115
7	Fracture	1	.276	.599

8	Ligament Rupture	1	.655	.418
9	Muscle Cramp	1	.000	.988
10	Muscle Pull	1	.301	.583
11	Puncture wound	1	2.951	.086
12	Sprain	1	12.980	.000
13	Strain	1	4.263	.039
14	Tendonitis	1	2.614	.106
15	Concussion	1	3.947	.047
16	Meniscus tear	1	1.947	.163
17	Low Back Pain	1	1.115	.291
18	Muscle Tear	1	1.960	.161
19	Rotator cuff	1	1.547	.214

The table 5-2 shows the association between injuries and game type. It was observed that association between Abrasion, Incision, Laceration, Sprain, Strain and Concussion and game type is high the value of χ^2 is higher than the table value. It shows that occurrence of these injuries and game types are not independent. In simple words we can says that these significant injuries have the higher probability of occurrence in team games in comparison of individual games.

4 CONCLUSIONS

After analysis the whole study following conclusion would be drawn:

- Abrasion and Sprain are more frequent and common injuries in team games.
- Muscle pull, contusion, sprain and fracture are most frequent injuries in individual games.

- Knee, ankle, and shoulder are most frequent and common body part which associated with injuries. Majority of injuries associated with the lower extremities in both the games. The leg is important in weight bearing part for speed in sport, subsequently the knee, ankle joints, foot, the muscles of the upper and lower legs are subjected to the greatest physical pressures that led to injury.

- The finger and wrist are easily injured in activities involving catching and holding of equipment in the events such as Kabaddi, Basket Ball, Badminton and in Hockey due to hit to fingers through a bouncing Ball.

- Preventive initiatives that focus on the sites of the body parts by sport are Cricket (Elbow, Shoulders, Fingers, Ankel, Thigh), Baseball (shoulder, ankle, hand, calf wrist), Kabaddi (knee, ankle, chin, elbow, fingers), Basketball (ankle, knee, elbow, shoulder), Hockey (knee, elbow, thigh, eyebrow, shin), Football (knee, ankle, thigh, calf, foot, elbow, shin and head), Wrestling (knee, elbow, fingers, ankle, ear and ribs), weight lifting (lumber vertebrae, palm, knee, thigh, shoulder), Badminton (knee, ankle, shoulder, elbow), Boxing (knuckles, nose, thumb, face, shoulder), Gymnastic (shoulder, hand, palm, knee, ankle), Judo (knee, face, ankle, shoulder, abdomen).

- Meniscus tear, ligament rupture, fracture, concussion and dislocation are most severe injuries found in various types of team and individual sports. Most of the injuries are minor, and moderate. Severe injuries are closely associated with highly stressful body contact and team sports such as, Boxing, Wrestling, Gymnastic, Basketball, Hockey, Football and Kabaddi.

- Percentages of match injuries are higher in team games and percentages of training injuries are higher in individual games.

- There is no significant difference found between new and recurrent injuries in team games and percentages of new injuries are higher in individual games.

- It is conclude that lack of knowledge towards sports injury and sport medicine may lead to recurrent injuries in various types of team and individual sports.
- Soft tissue injuries are most common and considered as minor injuries. The frequencies of soft tissue injuries are higher among all injuries in team and individual sports. Individual games have slightly higher frequencies in bone and joint injuries.
- Clay and grass courts are highly injury prone surfaces in various team and individual games and wooden surface was is considered as lowest injury prone surface.
- Improper warming-up, twist, fitness and jerk are most common intrinsic reasons in both team and individual sports.
- It is observed that most of the respondents do not know the exact reason of injuries occurred.
- Collision/Impact, fall or slip, field or playground, poor technique and unknown are the most frequent and common extrinsic reasons in various team and individual sports.
- The present study indicate that association between Abrasion, Incision, Laceration, Sprain, Strain and Concussion and game type are high. Except these injuries all other injuries and game type are independent mean there is no association between the occurrence of these injuries and game type.

5   RECOMMENDATIONS

This study conducted between team and individual sports competition. It is hoped that all the sports departments in India should come forward to adopt sports injury reporting system for documentation and for future research.

The resultant recommendations have been categorized as general prevention method of injuries in sports, and specific preventive methods.

5.1 General Methods of Preventions

The general recommendations have been classified as follow:

Physical Fitness

Good physical fitness is of the eventual important in dodging sports injuries. Whose basic physical fitness level is below normal are more prone to injuries. Regular exercise and general physical activities throughout the year can achieve a basic physical fitness level. General acclimatizing and training of large muscle groups is of great importance in most of the sports.

Warming-up and Cooling-down

The purposes behind warm up exercises are increase our range of motion of our joint and elasticity of our muscles which reduces the injury probability. Warm up increase muscle temperature, alertness and psychological preparation for the activity.

Cool down is also important as warming up which help a players in recover fast and washout the waste product after exercise.

Sports surfaces

It was observed that most common injury reason were impact, and fall or slip as we analyzed earlier in 4th chapter of this thesis. Quality sports surfaces reduce the slippery movement and improved cushioning especially landing from vertical movements. Most of the surfaces related to injuries were not well maintained.

Protective Equipment in Injury Prevention

A protective gear helps in reducing the chance of injury occurrence. But several factors affect the selection of protective gears. A protective gear is only effective when it meets the desired demands. It should be properly fitted. It should be made temperature absorbing material.

Knowledge of Rules
If a sportsperson follow the norms and standards made by the concerned authority he/she may certainly reduce the injury chance. It is only observation we have no any publication till now that knowledge of rules decrease the chance of injuries.

5.2 Specific injury prevalence methods

Injury Surveillance system
Information about the occurrences, nature of sports injuries and consciousness is the main product of injury surveillance. Injury surveillance is the first step in classifying the problem. Surveillance of injuries also helps in recognizing the cause of injuries so that injury prevention dealings can be developed as an intervention. This will permit for some injuries to be prevented. It is hoped that the coaches, administrators should appliance sports injury data collection system in their establishments that will help to develop injury prevention methodologies in all sports.

Curriculum Recommendation
New leanings in sports specific injury avoidance information be made accessible to referees, umpires, officials, coaches, Directors, teachers, players and parents about the nature and prevalence of sports injuries. Sports medicine should be a subjects in school or college students in their curriculum.

TABLE OF CONTENTS

Chapter- I

INTRODUCTION

Chapter-I

INTORDUCTION

Overview

Chapter-I

INTRODUCTION

I.   Introduction

A huge number of individuals around the globe partake in sports and physical exercises, at various levels, all the time. Games and physical movement of any sort are typically viewed as valuable for the person and in addition society overall, as a specific measure of activity is an imperative component in wellbeing advancement.

The potential risk for injuries in sports seem to increase for all level of athletes with increasing participation, intensity and demands as well as longer training periods. The severity of injuries is most commonly minor, moderate and severe in nature. In spite of this, injuries cost society billions of rupees in either direct or indirect costs. Besides, the competitors and additionally the group regularly encounter damage as a debacle. The incidence of injury levels need to be reduced and can be achieved by focused more on preventive measure. Through the years has been some interest in prevention. The sports community itself, by developing protective equipment, helmets, face masks and rule changes, has tried many ways to prevent injuries. In limited areas there has been some success, but more work needs to be done and a wide-ranging approach developed.

It is becoming progressively seeming that as well as having a health-giving aspect, sports can present jeopardy to health in the forms of accidents and harms. A person who needs to surrender or chop down his or her brandishing exercises because of game injuries can't a few or the greater part of his or her objectives. If the injury is serious enough the individual will also have resource to the medical services to be treated. Lastly, injury can result in absence from school or work.

I.1.1   History of Sports

For obvious reasons we do not know much more about athletic activities during the Stone Age. People probably liked games and plays, and they sang and danced. There is certain proof in sculptures, reliefs, and painting some 5000 years old that Egyptians exercised. The hieroglyphic sign for swimming dates from the same period.

It isn't until the point that the Olympic Games started that the historical backdrop of sorted out athletic exercises can be uncovered. While the derivation of the Olympic Games is not known exactly, there is an historical record of the ancient games beginning in Olympia in the western Peloponnese's, Greece, in 776 B.C. There after they were held at 4-years intervals, until AD 394 when they were abolished. There are numerous traditional clarifications of the origin of the game. One points the festival to Heracles, the most famous Greek hero. In art and literature he is represented as an extremely strong man of moderate height, a huge eater and drinker, very ardent, and generally kind but with occasional outbursts of brutal rage. This great fighter and hunter is famous for the Twelve Labours, or Dodekathlos, which include the capture of the lion Nemea, the cleansing of the stables of Avgeias in Elis, the capture of the Cretan Bull, and seizing the cattle of Geryon. Another myth tells us that there was a chariot race between Pelops and king Oenomaus, who used to challenge the suitors of his daughter Hippodameia. Pelops successfully persuaded Oenomaus servant to remove the wheel spindle pins: the chariot crashed and the king was killed. Unfair play is not a modern phenomenon in sports. Pelops married Hippodameia and become king of Pisa. He conquered Olympia where, for the glory of Zeus, he arranged competitions.

The earlier Olympic Programmes consisted almost exclusively of exercise of the Spartan type, testing endurance and strength with a special view of war. Later, more and more events were added: chariot races and horse races, wrestling and boxing, and the pentathlon including long jumping, quoit (discus) throwing, Javelin throwing, running and wrestling. Winners become national heroes; musicians sang their praises and sculptures preserved their strength and beauty in marble.

Olympia became an appearance of the Greek philosophies that the body of man further as his mental power and spar features a glory, that the body and mind ought to alike be disciplined, which it's by the harmonious discipline of each that men best honor of god Zeus. It ought to be noted that girls weren't allowed as competitors or, aside from the priestesses of Greek deity, as spectators.

Baron Pierre de Coubertin took the initiative of reviving the Olympic Games for athletes of all countries of the world, regardless of national rivalries, jealousies, and differences of all kinds, and with all consideration of all politics, race, religion, wealth and social status eliminated. An enthuastic conference at the Sorbonne, Paris, in 1894, It was decided that the games of the first Olympiad of the modern cycle should take place in Athens in 1896. However, we know too well that at times the high ideals expressed by Pierre de Coubertin have been neglected. **(Harries, 1994)**

I.1.2 Modern Organized Sports

Many sports have their origins in games contend with and while not balls and instrumentation enjoyed throughout the center ages and later. Preparation for looking, war, and defense created coaching in sport, Javelin throwing, fencing, shooting, boxing, and wrestling necessary for survival. Throughout the center ages the knights' tournaments were oft life and death struggles. Many historian claims that Great British were the founder of organized sports and at the start of the nineteenth century sports were introduced in class, and within the middle of the century championships were organized at faculties and universities and competitions befell between them, let's say the famed race between Oxford and Cambridge. In 1880 British Amateur Athletic Association was supported. As mentioned above than many few later Baron Coubertin launched the flagship of sport, the Olympic Games. **(Harries, 1994)**

An athletic injury is a medical resulting from activity that causes a limitation or restriction on participation in that activity, or for which medical treatment was received. Athletic injuries may stem from a single traumatic episode or form repeated overuse of a body part. For epidemiologic purpose, the inability to participate in a free, unrestricted manner defines athletic injury. The criteria for safe participation (and return to play following injury) include the ability to protect oneself during the sports activity.

The definition of injury thus hinges primarily on missed practices and game or participation in a limited fashion (no contact, no jumping, no cutting etc.). a quarterback laryngitis would be unable to participate, but no other team member would be affected by having this ailment. Likewise this narrow definition, a sprinter who falls and fractures his wrist after crossing the finish line during the last race of the day and who is able to participate without restriction the nest day after his arm is x-rayed and casted would not be listed as "injured". For this reason, another aspect considered in defining, an athletic

3

injury is when a "sentinel event" occurs, i.e., an injury that is significant regardless of its impact on one's participation status.

When athletic injuries are studied for epidemiologic purpose, the sensitivity of the definition of injury is a vital deliberation. Some studies consider the position of the athlete in the end of the training or game to conclude whether a reportable injury has happened **(Garrick JG, 1978)**.

They not include the time loss resulting from the initial sideline examination and management. Any athlete who is able to return to play without restriction prior to the end of the training or game is not considered to have experienced a reportable injury. Certain athletes may be recorded or may use additional protective equipment, thus allowing unrestricted participation. In these cases, the need for ongoing medical evaluation or treatment may later qualify this episode as a reportable injury. Other studies seek to eliminate minor or nuisance injuries from consideration. (Vinger PF, 1986) Their less sensitive definition counts only those injuries that result in restriction or limitation the next time there is a game or practice. This usually means the next day, but such is not always the case. Athletes injured on Friday evening in high school sports, for example, do not practice again until Monday. Similarly, athletes injured just prior to a holiday or vacation may not have their injuries counted.

Many athletes participate despite injuries, because they are willing to accept a less then optimal physical condition as a criterion for return to play. In his long and glorious professional football career, Walter Payton missed only one game of almost 200, and he claim he could have played in that one, too. It is hardly conceivably that he played professional football for over a decade and never experienced an injury. Similarly, athletes with chronic overuse conditions try to continue playing rather than succumb to the need for treatment and rehabilitation. In order to be able to study the epidemiology of injury, it is imperative that a clear definition of injury be established and that standard for safe participation is determined. **(Carol C. Teitz, 1989)**

I.1.3   Historical Perspective of Sports Medicine

In the Ayur-veda, medical manuscript of ancient India dating between 800 and 100 B.C., exercise and massage are recommended for chronic rheumatism. No doubt there were many prescriptions of this sort in earlier times since games and sports had been well known for many centuries and physical exercises to prepare for many centuries and physical exercises to prepare for military combat had already been systematized, but this is the first written record of this sort that has been preserved for us.

480 B.C. Harodicus was the ancient Greek writer whose works have survived to acclaim therapeutic exercise. He was a gymnast, one of the three classes of medical practitioners of ancient Greece. His prescriptions of exercise for the sick were so energetic that he was criticized by his existing Hippocrates in his many works.

460 B.C. Hippocrates made several references to the worth of physical activity, recommending it even for mental diseases, Herophilus and Eristratus, who taught at the medical school of Alexandria in the 4th span (century) B.C. both recommended moderate exercise.

126-68 B.C. Asclepiades was the 1st of the Greek physicians to practice in Rome. He treated his patients with different diets and by massage and recommended moderate exercise including walking and running.

About 25 B.C. Celsus advise frequent and vigorous exercise for hemiplegia, heart disease accompanied by failure, tuberculosis, and mental disease.

98-117 A.D. Rufus of Ephesus described the differing characteristics of the pulse in health and disease and its direct relationship to the apical beat of the heart.

130-201 A.D. Galen classified exercise for therapeutic purposes and recommended their use in moderation for many from of disease. He made and recorded more fundamental contribution to exercise physiology than any physician before or since. He was the first to develop systematic descriptions of the human body. He was the first to recognize that muscle has only one action, i.e. contraction. He observed that each muscle had only one direction of action and noted the antagonistic action of different muscle groups. He identified the stimulus to muscle contraction as coming from the brain via nerves. He described the connections and functions of the arteries and veins and showed that arteries contained blood obtained from the right side of the heart and air from the lungs. He described the formation of urine from the serous portion of the blood. He established the conception of tonus of a broad physical inspection and history taking based on logical principles. His influence was justly felt in medicine for over a thousand years.

With an advent of Galen we also come to the first known sports team physician. While practicing in Pregame following his return from Rome, he was entrusted with the care of the gladiators who performed in the public exhibitions. Through this work he developed his knowledge of anatomy and his skill in surgery.

Fifth century A.D.Akrelianus elaborated on the practice of medical rehabilitation including the use of hydrotherapy and of weights and pulleys. He was the first writer to recommend exercise during convalescence from surgery.

Seven century A.D.Paulus Aegineta recommended exercise and defined it as violent motion that renders body organs fit for their functional action.

Beginning of the tenth century The Arabic physicians translated the works of Greeks and Roman physicians, adding their own observation and recommendation.

About A.D. 980 Ibn Sina, followed the concept of Galen that medical gymnastics should include all healthful and health furthering exercise. During convalescence he advocated rest, baths, and gentle massgage. Since his influence remained great for centuries after his death, physicians of the middle ages advised against violent over activity in exercise and therefore against very vigorous sports and professional athletics.

1370-1444 Awareness was build up in medical gymnastics in Europe throughout the Resurgence by the reawakening of the original Greek contributions. Vergerius professor of logic at this University of Pauda, was one of the first Italian humanists to advocate the inclusion of regular physical exercise in the education of children. He influenced his contemporaries.

1378-1446 Vittorine da Feltre, who established under his partron, the Marguis Gonzango of Mantua, a school for the children of the court. They entered at the age of four or five, were tested for their capabilities, and then suggested exercises prescribed individually according to body type, age season, and time of the day. Dietetics was practiced and a wide variety of sports was employed. Gymnastics was conceived of as an integral and indispensable preliminary for educational success of the first time since ancient Greece. This development had influenced the course of education in the western world even since.

1407-1458 Maffeus Vegius believed in the obligatory introduction into education of gymnastics to strengthen the body and of sports for recreation. The 1st published manuscript on exercise by a physician was published in 1553 in Spain by Dr. Christobal Mendez of Jaen. He promoted exercise for older persons and for those who were crippled as well. He wrote "the easiest way of all to preserve and restore health without diverse peculiarities and with greater profit than all other measures put together is to exercise well". His book had apparently very little circulation and was discovered only recently.

1530-1608 A landmark of the sixteenth century was the publication in 1569 of the six books on the art of gymnastics by Gerola Mo Mercuriale. This work was written in popular style I order to appeal to a more general public than physicians. Mercuriale classified gymnastics into preventive and therapeutic forms but warned against strenuous military exercises and athletics. Ambroise Pare, in the introduction to his Surgery, referred to the doctrine of Galen that the body needs exercise for health. He prescribed different exercises for different types of persons and for different purpose. He felt that exercise of the limbs after the primary treatment of fractures was indispensable.

1529-1583 Laurent Joubert, professor of medicine at the University of Montpellier, was a great advocate of daily exercise. He considered physicians to be the only persons capable of prescribing gymnastics. He introduced therapeutic gymnastics into the medical course.

1546-1609 Joseph Duchesre wrote on exercise in his Ars Medica Hermitica, "The essential purpose of gymnastics for the body is its deliverance from superfluous humours, the regulation of digestion, the consolidation of the heart and the joints, the,

7

opening of the pores of the ski and the stronger circulation of blood in the lungs by strenuous breathing". He was the first to recommend swimming for strengthen the body as well as for the purpose of life saving, although the Spanish Physician, P.E. Gualtero, preceded his posthumous publication in 1648 by four years with an essay entitled. "Considerations to settle all doubts about the convenience of the art of swimming in order to keep health".

1543-1612 Marsilius Cagnatus of Verons in his preservation of health asked for specially educated physicians to supervise games and rowing into gymnastics.

1561-1636 Santorio, close friend of Galieo in Padua, invented the weighing chair, which enabled him to measure insensible perspiration and helped him to develop a basic theory of metabolic balance.

With the development of physiology and the study of mechanics, a new interest in animal and human movement became apparent. Jean Canape introduced a new era in exercise physiology with the publication of his essay.

1501-1576 Girolame Cardano the physician mathematician conceived a theory of muscle movement from a mechanical standpoint that exerted a profound influence on the physiologists of the next century.

Seventeenth Century The publication of work by Aldrovandi (on Quadripeds) in 1616 and Fabricius ab Aquanpendente (movement of animals) in 1614 ushered in the seventeenth century and paved the way for the work of Borelli.

1618-1679 Great Borellia Iatromechanical physiologist applied an understanding of mechanics and physical principles to the interpretation of all muscular action. He described muscular tone and the antagonistic actions of muscles, accepted the concept of innervation of muscles through nervous impulses, and failed inly in identifying the mechanism of contraction as a rearrangement of existing structure. His great work, on the movement of animals, was not published till his death.

1633-1714 Bernardine Romazzini wrote the first treatise of occupational disease. He pointed out that sedentary workers suffer from ill health and recommended regular exercise for them. Hoffman and Stahl as Halle wrote and lectured on the virtues of exercise in the prevention as well as the treatment of disease. Hoffman classified occupational movements as exercise, influencing Tissot, who, in 1780 produced his Medical and Surgical Gymnastics, one of the most influential books of its time. Tissot, who became surgeon-in-chief of the French army in 1808, prescribed exercises for their general effect, for strengthening muscles and moving joints. He founded, essentially, occupational and recreational therapy and adaptive sports. He advocated chest exercises to improve pulmonary capacity. Above all, he opposed prolonged bed rest.

Middle of the eighteenth century Nicholas Andry published his L'Orthospedie, which gave the speciality of orthopedics its name. He prescribed a variety of exercises for the prevention and treatment of diseases in children. He recommended exercise and sports as the means of alleviating and curing many infirmities and for reducing weight. Piere Jean Burette was the first physician to write on the history of sports, especially ball games and discus throwing.

In Russia, the first stirrings of interest in therapeutic exercise appeared in the seventeenth century. It was recommended to the Czar by his physicians that he should walk, run, and ride horse-back to correct his obesity. A.P. Protasov lectured in 1765 on the "The Importance of Motion in the Maintenance of Health". Twenty years later N.M. Ambodik wrote, "A Body without Motion Deteriorates and Purifies like Still Water".

In great Britain Robert Whytt, a neurologist of Edinburgh established that reflex action was mediated through the spinal cord. He understood fully the mechanism and significance of reflex action in games.

Beginning of the Nineteenth Century With the beginning of the nineteenth century, under the influence of ling from Sweden, Nachtegall in Copenhagen Clias in Berne, Jahn in Prussia, and Amoros in Paris, a true physical education apart from therapeutic exercise and no longer under medical direction was born. Ling introduced system into exercise. He based his method on what he called semi-active and semi-passive resistance exercise. George Taylor introduced the Ling System into America, where it became very popular.

Although machines for exercise had already been developed several hundred years ago, the enthusiasm for the Ling system became so great that not enough gymnastics teachers could be supplied. Zander supplied the demand with machines embodying levers, wheels, and weights for active, assisted and resistive exercise and massage, which soon became popular all over the world. Special hospitals were built in St. Petersburg and Moscow by Swedish gymnastics for the treatment of different illnesses. On the other hand, P.F. Lesgaft and W.W. Gorinewsky criticized the principles of Swedish gymnastics and showed that they were not in accord with anatomical and physiological principles.

1813-1878 Claude Bernard showed that the body performs a physiological synthesis by breaking down chemicals and building up complex substances. He also discovered the vasoconstrictor nerves.

1806-1875 Guillaume Duchesne de Boulogne, as a result of careful and detailed studies of striated muscle, comes to the conclusion that contraction of single muscle was not a normal occurrence.

1835-1911 John-Haughlings Jackson developed the concept of the hierarchy of levels in the central nervous system. He described it as a mechanism for the co-ordination of impressions and movements. Wars have always exerted social and economic consequences beyond their political significance. In modern times they have been a leading factor in stimulating the development of rehabilitative methods and services.

1898 The first English publication in Sports Medicine appeared in 1898 as a section on first aid in the Encyclopedia of sports and was written by J.B. Byles and Samuel Osborn, describing practical measures of emergency treatment for haemorrhage, wounds, bites, bruies, fractures, dislocations, strains, and head injuries and transportation for the injured person. It describes injuries commonly sustained in angling, boxing, cricket, football, hunting, lawn tennis, mountaineering, rowing and shooting and their management.

1910 Dr. Siefried Weissbein of Berlin produced a two volume work that he called 'Hygiene des sports' which is probably the first look to deal comprehensively with what we now call sports medicine. He described in his first volume the effects of sports activity as the function of the various organ system of the body and also discussed problems of clothing in sports and first aid for sports injuries of the commonly practiced sports of the day. He wrote separate chapters on games and sports suitable for children, women and elderly persons. This publication was followed in 1914 by Dr. G. Van Saar's one volume contribution to the Encyclopedia of Surgery, edited by Professor P. Van Bruns of Tabingen. This volume, entitled "Die Sportverlezungen,"dealt almost exclusively with injuries characteristics of certain sports and their treatment. In 1925, Dr. Flix Mandel published a work on the surgery of sports injuries.

Robert W. Lovett, an orthopedic surgeon of Boston, after treatment of patients of the first severe poliomyelitis epidemic in the United States, wrote that "muscle training constitutes the most important of the early therapeutic measure". Arvedson of Sweden also acknowledged the value of exercise in this as well as other musculoskeletal disorders. He pointed out to neurologist that destruction of cells in the cord was not complete and that the maintenance of muscle tone and the prevention of contractures were necessary to preserve any function that might remain.A revival of interest in underwater therapeutic exercise resulted partly from the contributions of Lowman, and Roen, Pope, and Hansson. Smith and Porritt introduced the use of suspension slings and spring-resistance exercise into therapeutic gymnastics.

1924 Burger proposed a series of positioning exercise to aid in vascular disease of the lower extremities. Twenty seven years later Veal et al. demonstrated the value of active and passive limb exercise in massive venous occlusion. A landmark of the study of exercise physiology was the publication of the Respiratory Function of the Blood by J.B. Rcroft.

1927 A general response to the leads offered by this pioneering work was delayed by the advent of World War 1. A.V. Hill of London delivered a series of lectures at the Lowell at Cornell University which were published as two monographs. Muscular movement in man discusses the factors governing speed and recovery from fatigue and introduces the concept of 'the steady state of exercise'. Living machinery describes the

11

relationship of neuromuscular co-ordination and cardiorespiratory function to strength, speed, and endurance.

F.A. Bainbridge's, "the physiology of Muscular Exercise" was published in its third edition in 1931, completely rewritten by A.V. Bock and D.B. Dill from the Fatigue Laboratory of Harvard University. It introduced the new concept of exercise physiology that had developed in Europe as well as at Harvard. All aspects of training and conditioning as understood at that time were discussed. The first edition of Edward C.Schnieder's Physiology of Muscular Activity appeared in the same year. Percy M. Dawson's physiology of physical education followed shortly afterward in 1935. All these works presented basic observation on exercise under a variety of conditions that have been proved remarkable accurate by subsequent investigations and that, in many instances, have not been much improved upto this time.

A revival of interest in muscular exercise as a means of physical rehabilitation and as a means of increasing strength occurred as the result of two publications following World War-II. Dr. Thomas Delorme published, with A.L. Watkins, "Progressive Resistance Exercise" in 1951. In carrying out rehabilitation of military personnel following surgery, he had applied his personal experience as a weight-lifter by giving them exercise against progressively increased resistance until they reached a maximum level or regained normal strength. Hettinger and Muller published their first work on isometric training in 1953, demonstrating that a maximum training effect could be achieved by a single daily isometric contraction maintained for only six seconds at two thirds of the muscle's maximum contraction strength. Although subsequent work in some laboratory indicated the increasing force of the isometric contraction to a maximum and the number of repetitions to between five and ten, and immediate world-wide valuable method to the use of progressive resistance exercise in training and rehabilitation. Credit for the first publication in English of works on sports medicine must be shared in England and America. C.B. Herald published "injuries and sports" in 1931. The first part of his work gives physiology of repair, first aid and emergency care, and physical therapy an applied to all sports injuries. In the second part, injuries to the various parts of the athlete's anatomy and their treatment were described in detail. Dr. Walter E.

Meanwell collaborated with the well-known football coach knute Rockne to produce the first American work in sports medicine. They discussed the relationship of the athletic trainer to problems of student health, the necessity of specialized training and the specific requirements, the responsibilities and duties of the team physician, the diet of the athletes, and the prevention and care of illness and injury in sports.

Publications all over the world in recent years have continued to expand our knowledge in sports medicine. These have included many volumes on physiology of exercise, athlete injuries, adaptive physical education, and subject related to interest. It would be unfair to mention some without a un-justice to other that might be intentionally or unintentionally omitted.

The preceding review does not pretend to be a comprehensive history of the origin and development of sports medicine, rather it is intended, by recalling what seems to have been some significant discoveries and contribution in the field of medicine and physical educations, to indicate that although sports medicine has achieved recognition as a particular discipline relatively, it has a historical background as ancient as any branch of those two fields and of greater age and tradition.

I.1.4 The international Federation and Sports Medicine
The first important attempt should be to bring together physicians interested in physical exercise and related problems, and to define as area of interest in sports medicine. It appears to have been the establishment of a separate section of "Hygiene of Physical Exercise" by Dr. A. Malwitz at the World Hygiene Exposition in Dresden in 1911. In March 1913, a medical congress dealing with sports was held in Paris, it dealt chiefly with physical therapy and the physiology of exercise. World War I brought an end to such meetings for a period of 15 years.

In February 14, 1928 during the second winter Olympic games at Saint Moritz, Switzerland, Drs. W. Knoll of Switzerland and F. Laterjet of France called together 33 physicians who have attending the team of 11 nations. This meeting established a committee whose function was to plan for the First International Congress of Sports Medicine to take place during the games of the IX Olympic at Amsterdam in August of the same year and to propose and plan an organization for a permanent international assembly of sports medicine. Dr.Mallwitz, Secretary and other members was Drs. Dybowski of Poland and Latarjet and Buytendijk of Holland.

When the congress met in Amsterdam, 281 physicians and specialists in physical education representing 20 different countries were present. The first Constitution of the Association International Medico-Sportive (AIMS) was adopted and F.J.J. Buytenkijk of Holland was elected President. Three principle purposes were included in the first constitution:

1. To inaugurate scientific research in biology, psychology and sociology in relation to sports.
2. To encourage the study of medical complications encountered in physical exercise in sports in collaboration with the various international sports federations, and
3. To establish international congresses on the area of sports medicine to be held throughout and at the site of the quadrennial Olympic games.

Although a physician from New York City named Brown was chosen to organize a congress at the X-Olympiad in Los Angeles in 1932, the meeting was never held, probably because no organized activities in sports medicine existed in the United State at that time. It was consequently agreed to hold the second congress at Turin, Italy in September 1933. By this time Dr. Laterjet was serving as President, following the resignation of Dr. Buytendijk. The topics discussed were grouped under nine headings: anthropology, charts for evaluating physical fitness, the medical control of sports, the kidney and the sports, respiratory physiology, fatigue, and women in sports. It was established that a general assembly of the new association would be held every four years at the time of the International Congress and its name was changed to the Federation International Medico-Sportive et Scientifique (FIMS)

I.1.5 Future Perspective of Sports Medicine
Through the world sports medicine is recognized as a specialty of medical practice. It is not well established in every country as yet, which might be expected because interest has crystallized recently. In every place where sports medicine has become well established it maintains a close relationship to those agencies and individuals who are

concerned with all aspects of the regulation of physical training, physical education, and sports. The establishment of centers for the medical control of sports has provided facilities and funds for research in sports medicine in which the persons engaged in these various disciplines may collaborate. Sports medicine has made and should continue to make important contributions to medical knowledge and practice. In therapy one must consider especially the contributions in therapeutic exercise or medical gymnastics that have come from the interest of physicians on sports and physical education. The earlier and more aggressive approach to the operative treatment of severe joint injuries is a direct outgrowth of experience derived from the care of athlete

At the same time, sports medicine has made contributions to physical education, among which is notably the development of adapted physical education. Through research in the physiology of exercise the way has been opened to improved performance in sports, especially in endurance events.

Finally, although great studies have occurred in the development of preventive medicine through sports medicine, in this area lays the greatest possibility for future achievements. Physical recreation will play an increasingly important part in the lives of the world's populations in the future. The steps taken so far by sports medicine to make it safe as well as enjoyable must be continued and greatly expanded. Although we believe that a lifetime of vigorous physical activity favors good health and longevity, the final and conclusive proof of this theory has yet to be made **(Pande, 1987)**

I.1.6 Sports Physiotherapy in India

Sports medicine in India is still in its infancy, so that sports physiotherapy as a part of the overall scope of sports medicine has not been very highly developed as yet, although it has already certainly made a significant contribution to the management of sports injuries. There are seven physiotherapy schools for basic training in India. Most of the courses last for two years, leading to a diploma or degree according to the school. Two schools, at Bombay and Baroda (Gujarat), have university-based courses lasting three years or slightly longer, leading to a degree. Sports medicine is included in the basic curriculum. However, there is no really specialized training in sports physiotherapy in Indian as yet, and there are very few jobs available within sports clubs or the sports federations. The board of control for cricket is one of the few bodies to employ physiotherapists. There for working at a sports center like the National Institute of Sports provide rare experience for Indian physiotherapists. The National Institute of Sports in Patiala is also the headquarter of the Indian Association of Sports Medicine (IASM). From time to time short courses are held there for doctors and physiotherapists who are mainly in general practice and who require orientation in the management of sports injuries. These courses are conducted by Indian expert in collaboration with visiting foreign experts, mainly from the Soviet Union an East and West Germany. In 1979, 26 doctors from 11 Asian countries attended the first three-week course in sports medicine at the National Institute of Sports in Patiala held under the aegis of the Federation International de Medicine Sportive (FIMS) and the International Olympic Committee (IOC), and leading to the Asian Diploma in Sports Medicine. In 1983, a three-week sports physiotherapy course conducted by the East German Expert Professor (Mrs) Helga Schmidt was attended by 31 physiotherapists and doctors. Since 1987, the National Institute of Sports has been running its own one-year diploma course in sports medicine. **(Grinsogono, 1989)**

I.1.7   Athletic Injuries
Injuries in sports due to acute distress or repetitive pressure related to athletic activities. Games wounds will affect bones or delicate tissue (tendons, muscles, ligaments). Consistently, a great deal of people (everything being equal) inside the world partake in physical activity and games exercises, from affiliation football field to softball jewels and Kabaddi courts. It's called playing at the same time, however wears exercises are more than play. Cooperation in sports enhances physical wellness, coordination and self-restraint, and give kids and individual profitable chances to learn collaboration. Amusement and games can likewise bring about wounds some minor, some genuine, and still others bringing about long lasting medicinal issues. **(Ajmer Singh, 2012)**

Sports carry an element of risk in the form of injury. In fact, there is no sport-whether amateur or professional-where injury does not occur. In some sports, chance injury may be much more due to the nature of the sport itself; in others, it may be less. The athletic injury may be as simple and insignificant as a bruise on the knee or elbow and as serious and fatal as a thigh fracture or skull smash. Athletic injuries occur from two different mechanisms: macrotruma, and microtruma. **Macrotrauma**-a deeply distressing experience-is a sudden injury from a major force. This could for example, be due to a bad fall from a horizontal (or parallel) bar or a ball hit during play in field hockey or cricket. Such situations abound in almost all sports, and can cause fractures, sprains or ligament, muscle strains (tear) and bruises or contusion, which are commonly termed as acute injuries. **Microtrauma** is due to repetitive injury over a long period of time and these injuries are also termed overuse. Types of injuries include stress fracture, little league elbow and shoulder impingement syndrome. Most sports injuries involve muscoskeletal system.

I.1.8   Health Risk of Steroid Abuse

There are many health risks from the use and abuse of anabolic steroids, Effects of anabolic steroid abuse on men include infertility, breast development, shrinking of the testicles, males pattern baldness, and severe acne and cysts. Effects of anabolic steroid abuse in women are: deeper voice, enlargement of the clitoris, excessive growth of body hair, male pattern baldness, and severe acne and cysts

Other effects of anabolic steroid abuse have been listed as delayed growth in adolescents, tendon rupture, increased LDL cholesterol, decreased HDL cholesterol, high blood pressure, heart attacks, enlargement of the heart's left ventricle, cancer, jaundice, fluid retention, HIV/ AIDS, hepatitis, "roid rage" - rage and aggression, mania, and delusions.

Athletes who use steroids can experience withdrawal symptoms when they quit, the symptoms include mood swings, depression, fatigue and irritability, loss of appetite, Insomnia, and aggression. Depression can even lead to suicide attempts, if untreated.

I.2   Statement of the Problem

The purpose of the present study was to compare the common sports injuries between team and individual sports. So, the study was entitled as "**A Comparative Study of Common Sports Injuries of Team and Individual Sports Competition**".

I.3 Objectives of the Study

After analysis the related literature available in the form of research articles, books, journals and other sources the following objective have been determined:

The following were the objectives of the study:

1. To study the descriptive profile of selected sample.
2. Percentage distribution, and injury ranking of common sports injuries of various team and individual sports.
3. Percentage distribution, of various body parts associated with injuries in team and individual games.
4. To study the injury severity of team and individual games based on total time loss due to injury.
5. To study the match and training injuries of team and individual games.
6. To study the new and recurrent injuries in team and individual games.
7. To study the type of injury (soft/bone/joint).
8. To study the different playfields and injury relationship.
9. To study the possible causes of injuries in team and individual games. (intrinsic and extrinsic)
10. To compare the ordinal data of sports injuries between the team and individual sports.
11. To prepare the three points grading of injury severity on normal distribution curve.

I.4 Delimitations of the study

The following were the delimitations of the study:

1. The study was delimited to team and individual sports person.
2. The study was delimited to male sports persons only.
3. The competition level of the respondents was delimited to Inter-University, National and International level.
4. The proposed study was delimited to the age group of 17-35 years.
5. The study was delimited to 300 subjects (N=300).

I.5   Limitations of the study

The following were the limitations of the study:

a) There were some factors which might have influenced the study like understanding level of the respondents, some medical terms used in the questionnaire and academic status of respondents.

I.6   Hypothesis of the study

It was hypothesized that:

- $H1_0$= **Occurrence of Abrasion and type of sports are independent** - there is no relationship.
- $H1_1$= **Occurrence of Abrasion and type of sports are not independent** - there is a relationship.
- $H2_0$= **Occurrence of Blisters and type of sports are independent** - there is no relationship.
- $H2_1$= **Occurrence of Blisters and type of sports are not independent** - there is a relationship.
- $H3_0$= **Occurrence of Contusion and type of sports are independent** - there is no relationship.
- $H3_1$= **Occurrence of Contusion and type of sports are not independent** - there is a relationship.
- $H4_0$= **Occurrence of Incision and type of sports are independent** - there is no relationship.
- $H4_1$= **Occurrence of Incision and type of sports are not independent** - there is a relationship.
- $H5_0$= **Occurrence of Laceration and type of sports are independent** - there is no relationship.
- $H5_1$= **Occurrence of Laceration and type of sports are not independent** - there is a relationship.

19

- $H6_0$= **Occurrence of Dislocation and type of sports are independent** - there is no relationship.
- $H6_1$= **Occurrence of Dislocation and type of sports are not independent** - there is a relationship.
- $H7_0$= **Occurrence of Fracture and type of sports are independent** - there is no relationship.
- $H7_1$= **Occurrence of Fracture and type of sports are not independent** - there is a relationship.
- $H8_0$= **Occurrence of Ligament Rupture and type of sports are independent** - there is no relationship.
- $H8_1$= **Occurrence of Ligament Rupture and type of sports are not independent** - there is a relationship.
- $H9_0$= **Occurrence of Muscle Cramp and type of sports are independent** - there is no relationship.
- $H9_1$= **Occurrence of Muscle Cramp and type of sports are not independent** - there is a relationship.
- $H10_0$= **Occurrence of Muscle Pull and type of sports are independent** - there is no relationship.
- $H10_1$= **Occurrence of Muscle Pull and type of sports are not independent** - there is a relationship.
- $H11_0$= **Occurrence of Puncture Wound and type of sports are independent** - there is no relationship.
- $H11_1$= **Occurrence of Puncture Wound and type of sports are not independent** - there is a relationship.
- $H12_0$= **Occurrence of Sprain and type of sports are independent** - there is no relationship.
- $H12_1$= **Occurrence of Sprain and type of sports are not independent** - there is a relationship.
- $H13_0$= **Occurrence of Strain and type of sports are independent** - there is no relationship.

- $H13_1$= **Occurrence of Strain and type of sports are not independent** - there is a relationship.
- $H14_0$= **Occurrence of Tendonitis and type of sports are independent** - there is no relationship.
- $H14_1$= **Occurrence of Tendonitis and type of sports are not independent** - there is a relationship.
- $H15_0$= **Occurrence of Concussion and type of sports are independent** - there is no relationship.
- $H15_1$= **Occurrence of Concussion and type of sports are not independent** - there is a relationship.
- $H16_0$= **Occurrence of Meniscus Tear and type of sports are independent** - there is no relationship.
- $H16_1$= **Occurrence of Meniscus Tear and type of sports are not independent** - there is a relationship.
- $H17_0$= **Occurrence of Back Pain and type of sports are independent** - there is no relationship.
- $H17_1$= **Occurrence of Back Pain and type of sports are not independent** - there is a relationship.
- $H18_0$= **Occurrence of Muscle Tear and type of sports are independent** - there is no relationship.
- $H18_1$= **Occurrence of Muscle Tear and type of sports are not independent** - there is a relationship.
- $H19_0$= **Occurrence of Rotator Cuff and type of sports are independent** - there is no relationship.
- $H19_1$= **Occurrence of Rotator Cuff and type of sports are not independent** - there is a relationship.

I.7 Definition and Explanation of the Terms Used

Extrinsic causes of sports injuries: these are the external causes of sports injuries for instance a collision with another athlete or by being struck by a piece of equipment used by an opposing player or teammate or equipment's/facilities/artifacts which are existing normally or abnormally in the sports environment/playfield gymnasium etc. **(Shaw & Gambhir, 2000)**

Intrinsic causes of sports injuries: these are the internal causes of sports injuries, for instance the health of an athlete or sports person, the physical and physiological state of locomotive organisms or tissues, pathological state of sports persons some infections or disease, poor fitness or fitness level, overload or chronic fatigue, improper training or training schedules, incorrect movement pattern or skill, or insufficient warming up/cooling down, lack of understanding about the games/sports/activity and their rules and regulation and psychological state of the sports persons etc. **(Shaw & Gambhir, 2000)**

Athlete foot: this is the tenia (fungus) infection of the toes. At initial sage condition cannot be recognized, but later, the skin between the toes thickness becomes white and causes itching. Infection can spread by common use of bath, showers, socks, and shoes. **(Shaw & Gambhir, 2000)**

Abrasion- a scraping injury to the skin. **(Griffith, 1989).**There is a partial loss of skin thickness. It may any grade of severity, from a simple excoriation of the skin by the opponent's headgear to very extensive damage. The major abrasion will occur over those parts of the body where there is a firm underlying tissue, particularly bone. Areas commonly injured are the shin, knee, iliac crest, elbow, and back of the hand. **(Vijay, 2001)**

Blister- Collection of the fluid in a "bubble" under the outer layer of skin. Blisters are overuse injuries of the skin. Due to friction, they are caused by mis-fitting shoes, a wrinkle in the sock, a foreign object such as a pebble in the shoe, or rubbing against an irregularity in the shoe itself. There is a focal point of irritation which feels "hot". Basically, a blister is a separated layer of skin with an accumulation of fluid. In cases where there is excessive friction, blood may form within the blister. There are usually more painful than the fluid-filled blister and are called blood blister. **(Wolpa, 1982)**

Contusion: A contusion may be defined a direct blow against the tissues, causing bruising of the skin or underlying tissues. This results in capillary rupture and an infiltrative type of bleeding, followed by edema and inflammatory reaction, and results into local swelling which may be superficial or deep depending upon the nature of the object striking and the location involved. **(Shaw & Gambhir, 2000)**

Bursitis: Bursitis is an inflammatory reaction within a bursa. It may vary in degree from very mile irritative synovitis with discomfort to suppurative bursitis with acute abscess formation. A bursa is specially formed to facilitate motion between contiguous layers of the body, and the athlete with his violence of motion is particularly prone to bursal involvement, resulting from repetitive local trauma due to tissue friction or from direct blows. **(Shaw & Gambhir, 2000)**

Dislocation: dislocation, or luxation, may be defined as an actual displacement of the opposing contiguous surfaces making up a joint, on presumes loss of function of some of the ligament structures of the joints, since the ligaments are designed to prevent displacement or abnormal motion. Subluxation is a partial dislocation. In acute sprain when the ligament finally tears, the joint subluxate either by a slipping of the bone ends on themselves or by a separation of the bone ends. If the force continues until the joint actually is disrupted, there is a dislocation. **(Khanna & Jayparkash, 1990)**

Fracture: A break in bone or ligament. Albeit for the most part a consequence of injury, a crack can be the after effect of a procured illness of bone, for example, osteoporosis, or of irregular development of bone in an innate sickness of bone, for example, osteogenesis imperfect ('weak bone infection'). Cracks are characterized by their character and area (for instance, greenstick break of the sweep). **(MedicineNet, 2017)**

Haematoma: A Haematoma will be defined as a collection of pooled blood within a relatively restricted area. Pooled blood is not blood which has infiltrated through soft tissues but rather blood which has collected in a localized and maintained its identity as blood. **(Shaw & Gambhir, 2000)**

Punctured Wound: This condition has been defined as a wound by a penetrating object, making a relatively small opening and continuing deeper into the soft tissues.

Sprain: a sprain is an injury to a ligament resulting from overstress which causes damage to the ligament fibers. Due to abnormal force the ligament becomes tense and then gives way at one or the other of its attachments in the substance of the ligament of a joint. It the attachment pulls loose with a fragment of bone, it is called a "**Sprain-Fracture**".

Strain: strain is defined a damage of some part or the unit (muscle, tendon, or the attachment) occasioned by overuse (chronic strain) or overstress (acute strain).

Stress Fracture: they are the common athletic injuries and should be considered when athlete complains of bone pain which is aggravated by activity and relieved by rest. Bone scan is very helpful in diagnosis of stress fractures.

Tendinitis: This is due to constant repetitive movements such as landing and jumping in Basketball, broad and high jump.

Tennis Elbow: It is characterized by pain and tenderness over lateral side of elbow. It is excessive amount of forearm rotation and gripping as in tennis and weightlifting. It usually subsides without treatment over a period of several months.

Chapter-II

REVIEW OF RELATED LITERATURE

Chapter-II

REVIEW OF RELATED LITERATURE

Overview

Chapter-II

REVIEW OF RELATED LITERATURE

II.   **Review of Related Literature**

Shashidhara,. & Krishnaswany, P.C, (2017). Conduct a study entitled "common sports injuries in athletics" the purpose of the study was to assess the common sports injuries in athletic. The term "sports injury," in its comprehensive sense, refers to the types of injuries that most usually occur during sports or physical activity. Accidents are also cause some injuries; others are due to poor working out practices, unsuitable equipment, lack of acclimatizing, or inadequate warm-up and stretching. Even though practically some part of your body can be wounded through sports or physical activity, the term is typically earmarked for injuries that involve the musculoskeletal structure, which includes the muscles, bones, and related tissues like cartilage. Athletic injuries my stem from a single traumatic episode or from repeated over-use of a body part. The status of the athlete at the end of the practice or competition to determine whether a reportable injury has occurred.

M, Umesh (2017). Title-"Rehabilitation of sports injuries through physiotherapy". The purpose of the study was to assess the effect of physiotherapy modalities on the pain of sportsperson of injury like sprain, strain, dislocation and other type of injuries which can distract the career of an individual. Thus the instrumentalize, healing treatment and guidance by the physiotherapist is necessary to get reduce of pain faster. The physically and mentally fit individual may present himself well in all undertakings, then the being unfit, hence the use of physiotherapeutic modalities such as electro gadgets use of therapeutic modalities have become most important in the modern sports. Physiotherapy is a partial relaxation treatment for injured and help for the further treatment.

In the study by **Balamrugun, K.V., & Bhat, K.V, (2017),** "entitled Prevalence and pattern of injuries among varsity basketball players". Objectives: to study the prevalence and the pattern of injuries of Inter-university Basketball Players. **Methods**: The study including 84 varsity basketball players (38 boys and 36 girls; with age range 17 – 28

25

years). Injuries to players during 2014–2016 seasons were registered by using a questionnaire. **Outcomes:** A total 68 sports injuries were documented with an incidence of 80.94 injuries per 100 athletes with the highest incidence being noted during competition and matches similar for male and female participants. Jumping/landing was the most common cause of injury (25%, N =17), followed by collision (20.50%, N = 14). Most of the injuries were at the lower extremities (62%, N = 42); with majority at the knee joint (26%, N = 18) and ankle/foot (19%, N = 13). Ligament sprain was the most common types of injury (41%, N = 28). Maximum of the injuries (N = 49, 72.6%) followed in the offensive half of the court and cryotherapy was the most frequently used managing modality to treat injuries. **Findings:** The overall incidence of injury among varsity basketball players was 80.95 injuries per 100 participants. The male gender revealed a greater risk of injury than the female players. Majority of the injuries were to the lower extremities and knee and ligament sprains were the most injury prone part of the body. Exercise-based injury avoidance Programmes planned to improve strength and neuromuscular control may help to decrease the occurrence of injuries.

Sandeep, U,. & Kuloor, H. (2017) designed a study entitled, "A comparative study on common injuries amongst the Greco roman and free style wrestlers among university wrestlers". **Objective:** The purpose of the study was to compare on common injuries between the wrestler Greco roman and free style wrestlers. **Methodology:** Total 50 wrestlers will be selected as subject, 25 wrestlers from both styles will be selected as subject randomly. As per the wrestlers response freestyle wrestling proved to be more injury prone than Greco Roman style of wrestling among the University wrestlers. Hence the researcher has taken up a study to find out injuries would take place during training and competition time in wrestler Greco roman and free style wrestler events among the players. The questionnaire administered consisting of questions related to common injuries (skin injuries, muscle injuries, bone injuries and joint injuries). The results of this study indicate that injuries are very common among the wrestler Greco roman and free style wrestlers. Results: It was concluded that players and coaches should be made more aware of the importance of protective equipment in helping to prevent injury or re-injury and effective emergency care of injuries by using rest, ice, compression and elevation. Majority of the Free Style wrestlers had Joint injuries. •

Majority of the Greco-Roman wrestlers had Muscle injuries. • By the outcome of this research hypothesis which was hypothized by the researcher has proved as null Hypothesis. • That is because usually freestyle wrestling involves quick movements and attacks on major parts of the body (upper and lower body) whereas in the Greco Roman wrestling only the upper body (above waist) is involved.

Kalra, S., Pla, S., & Pawaria, S. (2017) conduct a study entitled, "Correlational study of chronic neck pain and hand grip strength in physiotherapy practitioners". **Objective**: Chronic Neck pain is the 2nd utmost predominant musculoskeletal disorder seen in Physiotherapists after Low Back Pain. Uncomfortable postures, movements while handling patients, lifting, shifting and mobilizing the patients have been found to be risk factors for prolonged neck pain in Physiotherapists. Physiotherapists need to have a good grip strength while mobilizing and treating patients. Chronic pain has been known to have a deleterious effect on muscle strength. The present study planned to find the relationship of neck pain as measured by Visual Analogue Scale (VAS), Neck Disability as measured by Neck Disability Index (NDI) with grip strength measured by hand held dynamometer in Kilogram (Unit). **Materials & Methods**: 40 Physiotherapists working/practicing in different hospitals, clinics with chronic neck were selected for the study using Convenience Random Sampling. Readings were taken for neck pain, Neck disability and hand grip strength. Result & Discussion: Results of the study showed a significant negative correlation between neck pain and grip strength(r-0.35684) and neck disability and grip strength (r-0.419).Based on the results it can be concluded that Physiotherapists with chronic neck pain had decreased grip strength. Interference with ability of Nervous system to activate hand muscle through Motor Units may cause a reduction in Grip Strength and Grip Endurance. More over fear avoidance response as seen in patients with chronic neck pain for fear of injury leads to disuse atrophy and reduction in capacity to generate and retain force.

Khot, A., & Hande, D. (2017) conducted a study entitled, "Outcome of conventional balance exercises and electronic balance board on aging individuals". **Objective**: to study the involuntary injury due to lack of balance in elderly individual. Fall is the external causes of involuntary injury. It is the most common protest in the old age individuals which is due to loss of balance. Exercise based recuperation intercession is successful in limiting parity unsteadiness and diminishing the danger of fall. **Objectives:** was to find out the effectiveness of Electronic Balance Board along with Conventional Balance Training (CBT) on the balance performance in the aged presons. 50 old aged subjects were selected as subjects for the study. Group A were given CBT and Group B were given Electronic Balance Board Training along with CBT for 3 weeks and the risk of fall and balance were measured pre and post intervention then Data analysis was done using paired sample 't' test. **Results**: there was a significant improvement observed in the Group B in comparasion to Group A. Conclusion was that electronic balance board along with CBT has significant effects on balance than conventional balance exercise in elder individuals.

(Simbak, 2017) Designed a study entitled, "Modified rehabilitation exercises to strengthen the gluteal muscles with a significant improvement in the lower back pain". **Objective**: to study the effect of different type of rehabilitative exercise on the strength of gluteal muscles. **Conclusion**: The rehabilitation practices which found from the investigations that had done before more suitable than others to control and in addition enhance the Gluteal muscles toughness and this examination might be of awesome help for physical advisors in choosing practices while advancing individuals with low back pain (LBP) from low-force practices for those that require far more muscle action. The Surface Electromyography (SEMG) can be used to recognize the particular workouts which more suitable to be able to strengthen muscles and manage pain.

(Pandey, 2017) Conducted a study entitled, "Prevention & management of specific sports injuries through Ayurveda". **objective of the study**: to study the methods of avoidance of injuries through Ayurveda in sports". During the course of sports activity sportsperson experiences shoulder pain, knee pain and back pain. In Ayurvedic classics, it is pointed out that Vata dosha is responsible for most of the bodily activity & the same is vitiated during the deranged activity or over use of particular joint, which is responsible for variety of pain specially confined to muscle, joint and ligaments. Sport injuries are a kind of traumatic diathesis in which Vata dosha is provoked that may leads to pain at the site of affliction. Such types of injuries need special care to protect the suffering body parts. Current treatment modalities in modern medicine are oral steroidal and non-steroidal anti-inflammatory drugs (NSAIDs), which have a high rate and probability of unbearable gastric side effects and other systemic side effects. So, there prolong use is not admissible in sportsperson. In this concern ancient Indian healing system, Ayurveda addresses various therapeutic techniques & medicaments that can help a lot to the sports person. In practice, there are different treatment modalities for injuries such as uses of drugs, dietetics as well as practices of rehabilitation through Abhyanga (medicated oily massage), and Swedana (medicated fomentation). Sthanika vasti therapy (localized medicated vasti) aids to pacify the vitiated Vata there by relieving the pain & stiffness. Besides, Ayurveda also advocates herbal paste (lepa) for external application in the affected areas aid temporarily relief along with diverse heat modalities along with special poultice made up of rice gruel with oil make the joint more stable & viable.

(Colby, 2017) Colby, MJ, Dawson, B, Heasman, J, Rogalski, B, Rosenberg, M, Lester, L, and Peeling, P. Individual player injury data were documented over 4 full seasons (2012-15) from one professional club. The rate of non-contact wounds was thought about over the preseason, pre-rivalry, and in-season stages to choose similar noncontact damage chance. Workload of preseason and individual (settled) damage hazard factors (age, past damage history) were joined into the examination. A far reaching approximating count with a parallel calculated capacity shaped conceivable hazard factors with noncontact damage for chosen stages over the yearly cycle.Chances proportions were computed to decide the relative damage chance. Low aggregate total detachments in late preseason (<108 km) and precompetition (76-88 km) periods were connected with through and through ($p \leq 0.05$) more important harm chance in the midst of the in-season arrange. In findings, these results propose that in preseason competition period players has higher risk of get injured, with low preseason cumulative workloads related with improved in-season injury risk. So, the emphasis should be on strength and conditioning to achieving at least reasonable training loads.

(Kalina & Mosler, 2017) conduct a study to find out the cause of sports injuries. Falls are one of fundamental driver of accidental wounds. Estimating danger of damage

29

caused by a fall is main premise in showing safe fall methods to lessen such hazard. There were a few examinations which measures danger of wounds caused by fall by helplessness trial of body wounds amid a fall (STBIDF). Every single accessible work which includes estimating members by STBIDF were gathered and screened. 527 members in 18 unique gatherings were tried. The most minimal marker were seen in gathering of karate competitors on cutting edge level (SBIDF = 0.2), while the most astounding worth were appeared by gathering of individuals with scholarly incapacity (SBIDF = 11.12). General danger of damage level of tried individuals is high. Lower chance is associated with physical movement and involvement in combative techniques. Higher danger of damage is associated with low physical action level and co-event of various types of inabilities.

(Leung & Smith, 2017) This study explore the rates of wounds in school-level rugby association players in Australia utilizing the accord articulation for rugby association wounds. Damage reconnaissance was led on 480 rugby players from 1 school in Queensland, Australia. Damage information were gathered utilizing paper-based damage recording frames amid the 8-week rugby season utilizing a "restorative consideration" damage definition. Altogether, 76 players supported at least one wounds, with a sum of 80 wounds recorded. The general damage rate was 31.8 wounds/1000 match player hours (95% CI, 25.4– 39.4). Blackout had an occurrence rate of 6.0/1000 match player hours (95% CI, 3.5– 9.6). The rate of upper appendage and lower appendage wounds were 9.1 and 9.9/1000 match player hours, separately (95% CI, 5.9– 13.5 and 6.6– 14.5). The more established age divisions had higher damage rates and most wounds happened while handling or being handled. The damage rates saw in this example of Australian school rugby association players gives guidance for future investigations to empower educated choices identifying with improvement of damage aversion programs at this level of rugby.

(Meurer, Silva, & Baroni, 2017) Objectives: to depict the physiotherapists discernments and the present practices for injury avoidance in first class football (soccer) clubs in Brazil. Design: Cross-sectional examination was received for show think about. Football clubs engaged with the Brazilian head association 2015. Primary result measures Physiotherapists addressed an organized survey. Results Most physiotherapists (~88%) were dynamic in configuration, testing and use of avoidance programs. Past damage, muscle awkwardness, weakness, hydration, wellness, eat less carbs, rest/rest and age were viewed as "essential" or "vital" damage hazard factors by all respondents. The strategies most normally used to recognize competitors' damage chance were: checking of biochemical markers (100% of groups), isokinetic dynamometry (81%), surveys (75%), utilitarian development screen (56%), fleximetry (56%) and level hop tests (50%).

Yang C., Lee E., Hwang EH., Kwon O, Lee, J.H. (2016) A survey was conducted by the Korean Medicine team on National Volleyball team. Korean sports medicine doctors completed a questionnaire which includes injury parameters such as type, location, situation and pain scores. Total 166 cases of injuries were reported out of 94 male and female Korean national Volleyball players. Highest frequent injuries were knee (25.9%), low back (13.3%), elbow and ankle (8.4%) respectively. Major injured tissues joints (41.6%) and muscles (30.7%) observed respectively. Following methods of Therapeutic modalities operated by KM team medical doctors: acupuncture (40.4%), Chuna manual therapy (16.00%), physical therapy (15.22%), taping (9.00%), and cupping (7.82%) for treating Volleyball injuries. The purpose of this study was to present the preliminary injury profile of elite Volleyball players of Korea. These parameters could be helpful to make advanced KM model in sports medicine. (Yang, 2016)

A.E, Mohammed, (2016) construct a study entitled, "Common Sports Injuries" **Objective**: to review the general common sports injuries. Consistently, many individuals everywhere throughout the world take part in amusements and games exercises or physical activity. Cooperation in sports enhances physical wellness and general wellbeing and health. Physical activity and games can likewise bring about wounds, some minor, some genuine and still other in long lasting medicinal issue. Games wounds result from intense injury or monotonous pressure related with athletic exercises. Games wounds can influence bones or delicate tissue (tendons, muscles, ligaments). There are various games wounds occurred in the field of games. It is critical for all mentors, coaches and players to know the causes side effects, counteractive

31

action and treatment for all these regular wounds with a specific end goal to maintain a strategic distance from the majority of these sorts of wounds, additionally to refresh the poor preparing techniques.

In 2016, Singh, K designed a study entitled, "Psychological strategies for faster injury recovery". Objective: to deal with the psychological strategies and there effect on healing from sports injuries. during the play players often have to undergo from injuries. For fast healing from sports injuries several type of physical strategies are accepted by the players but mental strategies are also important side by side. But players often pay no attention to them. This slows the process of recovery and healing process of mental as well as physically.

BS, V.M, (2016) organized a study entitled, "Common injuries in Kabaddi player and their prevention with the help of biomechanics". Objective: to review present research on importance of biomechanics in preventing sports injuries and to present biomechanics applications related to Kabaddi technique, Kabaddi play and concepts of injury avoidance. With the help of biomechanics upgrading of skill used by teacher and coaches to correct motion and techniques of an individuals. Furthermore, researchers in the arena of biomechanics may develop a new and more effective technique for better execution of a sport motion. Some important aspects related to common injuries during Kabaddi playing and their prevention with the help of biomechanics is discussed. Conclusions are drawn based on the qualitative analysis.

A.N., Mohammed, & Dhinu, M.R., (2016) designed a study entitled, "Assessing common epidemiology among university male boxers". Objective: to assess the common sports injuries among intercollegiate level male boxers. Methodology: A total of sixty (N=60) inter collegiate level male boxers in different colleges from the Calicut University were selected as subjects and their age ranged from 17 to 22 years. The subjects had represented the college at least once in intercollegiate level competitions. The present study was based on common injuries to the players and their causes, reasons, method of treatment to injuries, other related aspects and personal profile. The data were collected through questionnaire and followed by personal interviews of the players. The percentage analysis was employed to analyze the incidence of common injuries. The following conclusions were drawn based on the results of the study. The majority of injuries occurred to the boxers were on upper extremities, head and faces. Subjects repeatedly got injuries at the same part and injuries occurred during both practice and competition sessions. Injuries affected the performance capacities of the players both physically and psychologically. Boxing requires a variety of physical attributes and specific playing skills. Participants should be trained to meet the physical, physiological and psychological requirements to cope with demands of play and reduce the risk of injury. It is recommended that the physical education teachers the coaches and the players should be given proper education and training with respect to the need for conditioning programs during practice sessions and the use of correct techniques during competitive boxing to avoid injuries.

(Pradeep T, 2016) Objective: To study the effect of combined dynamic hamstring and quadriceps stretching on knee joint position sense. Method: 15 healthy individuals randomly assigned in to three groups. Every cluster go through dynamic quadriceps stretch, hamstring stretch and combined quadriceps & hamstring stretch. Absolute angular were measure through Shadow goniometer at 70o. **Outcomes**: The investigation of pre and post extend Absolute precise mistake inside gathering uncovers that it was factually critical inside joined gathering (p<.012), hamstring (p<.005) than quadriceps gathering (p>.378). Anyway examination between bunch uncovered that, the investigation of fluctuation between three gathering after intercession i.e. consolidated (2.47±1.60), Hamstring (1.93±1.44) and Quadriceps (4.80±3.30) was observed to be factually huge with (p <.003). Conclusion: It is inferred that dynamic extending of hamstrings or consolidated stretch (quadriceps and hamstring) has noteworthy impact on enhancing knee JPS contrasted with quadriceps alone in sound grown-ups when estimations were taken in knee flexion development.

(Khatun, 2016) Conduct a study entitled, "A study of selected sports injuries and their preventive and rehabilitative measures among women soccer players of west Bengal soccer clubs". Objective: to study the sports injuries and their preventive and rehabilitative measure among women soccer players from the clubs of West Bengal. The purpose of the study was to study of selected sports injuries and their preventive measures among women soccer players of West Bengal soccer clubs. The subjects for this study were one hundred sixty eight women soccer players, coaches, assistant coaches and doctors of eight West Bengal soccer clubs. The variables selected for this study were sprain, strain, contusion, abrasion, dislocation and fracture. A set of thirty five questions for soccer players and fifteen questions for coaches and doctors was constructed for collection of data. Percentage analysis was employed for analysis of data. The result shows that Women soccer players of West Bengal mostly suffered from bone injury followed by muscle injury and joint injury. This might have the reason for aggressive tackling by players or foul play. Treatments and its managements in selected soccer clubs revealed the facts that good percentage of injured players were referred to specialist but players faced economic strain for their treatment. In most of the injury cases physiotherapy was the commonest mode of treatment. To prevent occurrence of soccer injuries good measures were taken by the players themselves, the coaches, the doctors and management itself. Results: However, the study revealed that 100% effort and supervision to avoid players' injuries were not provided. As a result a gross percentage of more than 40% of players were left without adequate prevention so far as knowledge and practice are concerned. This might be due to the lack of emphasis on precautionary measures and continuous supervision by the concerned personal as well as the education of the players themselves. So far as awareness and education of women soccer players about injuries are concerned, it was revealed that inspite of being the member of soccer clubs of West Bengal 100% of their players were not aware of sports injuries.

(Kuzuhara, Shibata, & Uchida, 2016) Background of the Study: Mini-basketball is one of the most popular junior sports in Japan. Mini-basketball-related injuries may increase because of early specialization. **Objectives**: To study the incidence rates, body part associated, classification, and mechanisms of sports injuries in mini-basketball teams. Design: Descriptive epidemiology study. Setting: Mini-basketball teams in Kobe, Japan. Patients or Other Participants: A total of 95 players in 7 community-based mini-basketball club teams (age range, 9 through 12 years). Main Outcome Measure(s): Data on all practice and game injuries for the 2013-2014 season were collected using an injury report form. Injury rates were calculated according to site, type, and mechanism. **Results**: The overall injury rate was 3.83 per 1000 athlete hours (AHs). The game injury rate (12.92/1000 AHs) was higher than the practice injury rate (3.13/1000 AHs; P < .05). The most common anatomical areas of injury during games and practices were the head and neck (36.4%, 4.70/1000 AHs) and the upper limbs (47.8%, 1.50/1000 AHs). Sprains (42.9%, n=39) were the most common type of injuries overall, followed by contusions (29.7%, n = 27). Most game injuries resulted from body contact (45.5%, 5.87/1000 AHs), whereas most practice injuries resulted from other contact (56.5%, 1.77/1000 AHs). **Conclusions**: rates of injuries during games were higher than rate of injuries during practice in Japanese mini-basketball players.

Guhane, T.F, (2015) This review provides the information about sports injuries with possible Causes, Symptoms, Treatment and Prevention. Exercising is good for you, but sometimes you can injure yourself when you play sports or exercise. Accidents, poor training practices, or improper gear can cause them. Not warming up or stretching enough can also lead to injuries.

(Pastor, Ezechieli, Classen, Kieffer, & Miltner, 2015) OBJECTIVE: The aim of the study was to examine prospectively over 6 seasons the acute and overuse injuries of a German male professional volleyball team. **METHODS:** The study included 34 male national league players from season the 2007/08 to 2012/13. All players received a sport medicine examination and a functional diagnosis before each season. Based on the results the players received an individual training plan. **RESULTS**: The players suffered 186 injuries. The prevalence of acute injuries was 1.94 per player and overuse injuries 0.64 per player. The incidence of acute injuries was 3.3/1000 h volleyball and overuse injuries 1.08/1000 h volleyball. The largest number of injuries was found in the spine. The players had most likely minor injuries. The players had significantly fewer injuries in their second season (1.92) than in their first season (3.25; p = 0.004). **CONCLUSION:** It could be concluded that volleyball is a sport with a relative low occurrence of injuries compared to other team sports. The prevalence of injury is 2.58 per player. Due to an injury a player dropped out 16.91 days per season. An individual training program seems to reduce the incidence of injury.

(Mazer, et al., 2010) OBJECTIVE: To pronounce the method of managing musculoskeletal injury in children and examine factors prompting return to play assessments with different health care professionals. **DESIGN:** National survey. **TOOL AND TECHNIQUES:** online questionnaire was used. **PARTICIPANTS:** doctors, physical therapists, and therapists of athletes who were members of their particular sport medicine specialty organizations. **Independent variables of the study:** Professional affiliation and the effect of the following factors were examined: parent, cautious parent, protective equipment, previous injury, musculoskeletal maturity, game importance, position played, team versus individual sport, and time since injury. **Main findings:** Commendation of return to activity after common injuries seen in children and youngsters as described in 5 vignettes; reliability of responses across vignettes. **RESULTS:** To accomplish the study 464 respondents (34%) were selected to complete the survey. There were numerous dissimilarities between the professional groups in their recommendations to return to activity. Most factors studied didn't tend to influence the choice to come back to activity, though protecting instrumentality usually inflated the response to come back sooner. The number of Participants who would return a child to activity sooner or later for each factor varied greatly across the 5 vignettes, except for pushy parent or cautious parent. **Conclusions:** Management practices of sport drugs clinicians vary per profession, child, clinical factors, and sport-related factors. Choices relating to come back to play vary per five specific characteristics of every clinical case. These findings facilitate establish areas of agreement and disagreement within the management of youngsters with injuries and safe come back to physical activity.

Schmikli, Sandor, L Msc, Backx, Frank, J G MD, Kemler, Helena J MSct. (2009) A national survey was conducted on sports injuries in the Netherlands. The main purpose of this study was to define populations for sport injury prevention programs and risk factor assessment: the type of age, gender, and game was designed to separate subgroups with adequate contributions to injuries. Sport sport participation was associated with 1.5 million injuries per 10,000 hours. 50% of these were to be treated medically. All of the medical treatment injuries were linked to 2/3 games. Age was classified as follows: Open-air football (male age 4-54 years and women of 4-17 years old), indoor football (men 18-34 years old), tennis (male / female 35-54 years) ,

Volleyball (female / 18-54), field hockey (18 to 34 years of age, 4 to 17 years of age) and race / jogging (men and women from 35 to 54). Found that the average cost of treatment was 400 million, respectively It was concluded that the survey identified the largest targeted population (sports, age and gender) for injury prevention programs in the Netherlands.(Schmikli, 2009)

(Spinks & McClure, 2007) Injuries due to sport and other forms of physical activity and exercise in young children represent a significant burden on public health. It is important to compute this risk to confirm that the potential benefits of involvement in sport do not outweigh the disadvantages. This review summarizes the literature that reports exposure-based injury rates for various forms of physical activity in children aged 15 or under. Forty-eight studies were found, of which 27 reported injury rates by measuring the time of exposure and 21 reported injury rates with another measure. Fourteen different sports and activities have been covered, mainly team sports, with football as the most studied sport. The definition of lesions and the method of determining and measuring lesions differed from study to study, which created a wide variation in reported injury rates that did not necessarily represent actual differences in the risk of injury between injuries and activities. The highest proportions of hourly injuries were recorded for ice hockey, and the lowest proportions were for football, although the range of injury rates for both activities was wide. Very few studies have examined sports-related injuries in children under the age of 8 or in unorganized sports situations.

(Hootman, Dick, & Agel, 2007) Objective: The National Collegium Athletic Association (NCAA) summarizes the 16-year injury data types in 15 sports and identify the potential risk factors that can prevent injury. **Background**: In 1982, the NCAA initiated gathering standardized injury and exposure data for collegiate sports through its Injury Surveillance System (ISS). This special issue reviews 182 000 injuries and somewhat more than 1 million exposure records captured over a 16-year time period (1988-1989 through 2003-2004). Injuries of practice and games that required medical care and lead to in at least 1 day of time loss were included. An exposure was defined as 1 athlete participating in 1 practice or game and is expressed as an athlete-exposure (AE). **Main Results**: Combining data for all sports, injury rates were statistically significantly higher in games (13.8 injuries per 1000 A-Es) than in practices (4.0 injuries per 1000 A-Es), and preseason practice injury rates (6.6 injuries per 1000 A-Es) were significantly higher than both in-season (2.3 injuries per 1000 A-Es) and postseason (1.4 injuries per 1000 A-Es) practice rates. No significant change in game or practice injury rates was observed during the 16 years. More than 50% of all injuries were associated with the lower extremity. Ankle ligament sprains were the most common injury over all sports, accounting for 15% of all reported injuries. Rates of concussions and anterior cruciate ligament injuries increased significantly (average annual increases of 7.0% and 1.3%, respectively) over the sample period. These trends may reflect improvements in identification of these injuries, especially for concussion, over time. Football had the highest injury rates for both practices (9.6 injuries per 1000 AEs) and games (35.9 injuries per 1000 A-Es), whereas men's baseball had the lowest rate in practice (1.9 injuries per 1000 A-Es) and women's softball had the lowest rate in games (4.3 injuries per 1000 A-Es). Recommendations: In general, participation in college athletics is safe, but these data indicate modifiable factors that, if addressed through injury prevention initiatives, may contribute to lower injury rates in collegiate sports.

(Murray, Murray, Mackenzie, & Coleman, 2005) OBJECTIVES: To study the diagnosis and management of adults attending a sports injury clinic to regulate how the management of the two most common injuries treated in this clinic is based on evidence and to explore factors that affect management. **METHODS**: A review examination of 100 arbitrary case notes separated age, sex, game, sort and site of damage, treatment, and result. Precise writing surveys inspected the degree and nature of logical proof for the administration of the two most generally introducing injuries. A clinical connection period and specialist interviews permitted acknowledgment of components impinging on administration choices. **RESULTS**: Patellofemoral pain syndrome (PFPS; 10% of all injuries) and Achilles tendinopathy (6% of all injuries) were the most commonly presenting injuries. The mean (SD) number of treatments used for PFPS was 2.8 (0.9). The mean number of treatments used for Achilles tendinopathy was 3.7 (1.0). Clinicians reported that personal experience formed the basis of management plans in 44% of PFPS cases and 59% of Achilles tendinopathy cases, and that primary research evidence only accounted for 24% of management plans in PFPS and 14% in Achilles tendinopathy. Professionals were uninformed of writing supporting more than half of the treatment modalities they utilized. Be that as it may, clinicians were regularly utilizing proof based medications, unconscious of the supporting exploration information. Determinations: This examination features an absence of proof base, an absence of learning of the exploration confirm, and an absence of administration in view of the present confirmation that is accessible for these conditions. Specialists rehearsed confirm based solution in less than half of cases.

(Kovacic & Bergfeld, 2005) OBJECTIVE: The sole purpose of this manuscript is to summary general treatment and return to play (RTP) tactics as they pertain to athletes with numerous upper extremity injuries: A review of the literature plus expert opinion served as the basis for recommendations made regarding management strategies for returning the athlete to play after upper extremity injury. A Medline search was performed using the following key words: upper extremity injury, return to play, glenohumeral dislocation, acromioclavicular joint sprains, elbow dislocation, scaphoid fracture, metacarpal fracture, finger dislocation, tendon injury, hand, mallet finger, and jersey finger. These and other related terms were crossed using the Medline database from 1966 to 2005. RESULTS: Survey of book parts, articles produced from the Medline hunt, and master feeling prompted the proposals that are exhibited here. There is general assention with respect to the treatment of a considerable lot of the wounds talked about, yet debates do exist. RTP rules are to a great extent subject to the seriousness of starting damage, rates of recuperating, and return of quality. Decisions: Each competitor with specific damage to the furthest point should be drawn nearer as a person as no single arrangement of treatment or RTP rules applies to all wounds or all people. Factors, for example, age, damage seriousness, hand predominance, kind of game interest, technique for treatment, and chronicity of damage are among the numerous issues that must be considered when building up a treatment and RTP system for a specific competitor.

R A Stretch has directed a study on cricket players of south Africa: OBJECTIVE: To define the incidence and nature of injuries persistent by elite cricketers during a three season period in order to identify possible injury patterns. METHODS: 36

physiotherapists and 13 therapeutic specialists in work with 11 provincial and the South African national groups finished damage reports shape for every cricketer who gave damage amid each season to decide anatomical site of damage, month of damage amid the season, finding, component of damage, regardless of whether it was a return of past damage, whether the damage had happened again amid the season, and historical information. **RESULTS:** A sum of 436 cricketers saw 812 wounds.bowlers (41.3%), handling and wicket keeping (28.6%), and batting (17.1%) represented the greater part of the wounds. The lower appendages (49.8%), upper appendages (23.3%), and back and trunk (22.8%) were most ordinarily harmed. The wounds happened basically amid five star matches (27.0%), constrained overs matches (26.9%), and hones (26.8%) amid the early piece of the season. Intense wounds made up 64.8% of the wounds. The more youthful players (up to 24 years) maintained 57% of the first run through wounds, and the players more than 24 years old managed 58.7% of the wounds that repeated from a past season. The wounds were chiefly delicate tissue wounds overwhelmingly to muscle (41.0%), joint (22.2%), ligament (13.2%), and tendon (6.2%). The essential instrument of damage was the conveyance and finish of the quick bowler (25.6%), abuse (18.3%), and handling (21.4%). **DECISION:** The outcomes show an example of reason for damage, with the youthful quick bowler well on the way to support intense damage to the delicate tissues of the lower appendage while taking an interest in matches and works on amid the early piece of the season.

Chapter-III

RESEARCH PROCEDURE AND METHODOLOGY

Chapter-III

RESEARCH PROCEDURE AND METHODOLOGY

Overview

CHAPTER-III

RESEARCH PROCEDURE AND METHODOLOGY

III. Research Procedure and Methodology

Injuries caused by participation in various games for sports are more common today since more people are involved in sports of all type. Many new and often high risk sports now exist, for example, hand gliding. The age range of competitors has widened with, children started sports, younger and adults continuing longer. Professional athlete need to be fitter today than those athletes in previous year. They compete more frequently and often at a higher level, as witnessed by the speed with which records fall.

In India, the sports, still is an upcoming field. Now a day the athletes are going towards professionalism. With this cause the standard of sports is also increasing and the level, nature and type of injuries among the Indian male athletes are increasing. So it is very important for the professional of physical education and sports to know the different kind of injuries among Indian male and female athletes. But the present study focuses on male athletes only.

The purpose of the study was to compare the common sports injuries in team and individual sports competition. An attempt had been made by the researcher to endure the dimensions of the injuries in team and individual sports competition by identifying the different aspects related to sports injuries.

This chapter describes the procedure adopted for selection of subjects (source of data), selection of variables, development of inventory, and administration of inventory, collection of data and statistical analysis of data.

III.1 Selection of the Subjects

As per the advises of the experts including my supervisor and prevailing practices, keeping in view the feasibility and purpose of the study, it was resolve to collect data from following sources.

41

- Sportspersons (Male only)
- Team Game
- Individual Game

Keeping in view the statistical guidelines and feasibility in mind the numbers of samples from each category were planned as per the advice of the statisticians. The detail descriptions of sources are explained in table: 3.1.

Table III-1 : Classification of Sample

GAME TYPE	SPORTS	SAMPLE (N)
	Cricket	25
	Baseball	25
	Kabaddi	25
	Basketball	25
Team Games	Hockey	25
	Football	25
	Total Subjects from Team Game	**150**
	Wrestling	25
	Weight Lifting	25
	Badminton	25
	Boxing	25
Individual	Gymnastic	25
Games	Judo	25
	Total Subjects from Individual game	**150**
	Grand Total (150+150)	**300**

From the population a total 300 samples were selected through random sampling technique from Team and Individual sports competition, out of the total sample half of the sample (N=150) were from team game and (N=150) were from individual game. Six games were selected for team game and Six games were selected for individual game (see table 3.1). 25 male sportsperson of national/inter-university/international from each delimited games were planned for sampling. The age of selected samples were ranged from 17 to 35 years.

III.2 Selection of Variables

The research scholar critically studies the available scientific literature from sport medicine books, journals, magazines and periodicals etc. related to sports injuries. As well as keeping in view the feasibility criteria, availability of the instruments, experts' opinion and the purpose of the present study following variables have been selected:

Under the objective of type, classification and distribution of common sports injuries following variables have been selected:

1. Common sports injuries
2. Body parts associated with sports injuries.
3. Time lost in days due to injury.
4. Injury occurred during match and training.
5. New and Recurrent injuries.
6. Injury type (soft, bone, and joint injuries)
7. playfields and injuries

Under the objective of sports injuries severity following variables have been selected:

1. Injury associated with the greatest time loss in team games.
2. Injury associated with the greatest time loss in individual games.
3. Injury associated with the greatest time loss in each selected game.

Under the objective of reasons of sports injuries following variables have been selected:

1. Intrinsic reasons of injuries
2. Extrinsic reasons of injuries

III.3 Development of Injury Report Inventory

The distinction and interpretation of sports injury statistics are relevant to role of athletic trainers, who are responsible, in part, for promoting the safety of sports in society. It is therefore important for athletic trainers in all setting to gain an understanding of the cause of and risk factors for sports related injury. To do this athlete's trainers must be able to accurately measure and assess injury related data. So, the development of injury inventory is a most important factor in sports injury research.

In order to gain knowledge about athletic injuries, it is necessary to record and report injuries. It is essential that those who report injuries be properly educated about the terms and definitions of injury, what information to gather, and how to record this information on the appropriate forms. There must be completeness, uniformity, accuracy, and standardization of methodology to be able to make meaningful comparisons among different reports of injuries.

A data collection system must consider exactly what information is to be gathered and who will record the data. The forms utilized must be appropriate for the task. All reporters should be carefully educated, clearly understanding and all terms and definitions. Completeness, accuracy, and uniformity are essential in conducting any injury study.

STEP-I Objectives of the Sports Injury Inventory

1. To study the demographic information of selected sample.
2. Percentage distribution, frequency distribution, percentage ranking of injuries in selected games.
3. Incidence rate, percentage distribution, frequency distribution and percentage ranking of body part associated of injuries in selected games.
4. Distribution of injury severity in relation to days lost from training and competition due to injury in selected games.
5. Assessment of match or training injuries.
6. Assessment of new and recurrent injuries.
7. To assess the type of injury (soft/bone/joint)

8. To assess the playfield and injury relationship.
9. To find out the possible reasons of injury (intrinsic and extrinsic)
10. Comparison of sports injuries between team and individual games.

STEP-II Selection of Item

1. Demographic information includes Name, Age, Height, Weight, Game, Playing Position, Gender, Region, Level of Competition, Playing Experience, Training Hours and University.
2. List down the injuries you have experienced due to your games/sports.
3. Body part associated with injuries.
4. Time lost in days (for obtained severity).
5. When Injury occurred? In Match or Training
6. Injury classification. (New and Recurrent Injuries)
7. Injury Type. (soft tissue, bone and joint injuries)
8. Type of playfield related to injury.
9. Possible causes of injury which are listed.

STEP-III   Development of Blue Print

Then the blue print was prepared comprising the above inventory, there after subjected for trail run.

STEP-IV   Trial Run

After the trial run few modifications were made based on the most commonly agreed language, inventory, questioning etc.

STEP-V   Reliability, Validity and Objectivity of the Inventory.

The developed inventory was obtained open ended responses. So, the inventory was considered sufficiently reliable and objective as it was designed under the guidance of number of experts by adopting phase wise trial run and followed by required improvement based on most commonly agreed language, presentation, nature of inventory, nature of questioning and required/responses to design the final shape of the inventory ultimately. Thus, keeping in view the feasibility, the statistical means of reliability were also established. As earlier said that the inventory consisted of open-ended responses so, following method of reliability were used:

Inter-Rater Reliability

In statistics, inter-rater reliability, inter-rater agreement, or concordance, is the degree of agreement among raters. It gives a score of how much consistency, or consent, there is in the ratings given by adjudicators, and it is one of the aspects of test validity. It is useful in refining the tools given to human judges, for example by determining if a particular scale is appropriate for determining a particular variable. If various raters do not agree, either the scale is defective or the raters need to be re-trained. There are a number of statistics which can be used to determine inter-rater reliability. Different statistics are appropriate for different types of measurement. Some options are: **joint-probability of agreement, Cohen's kappa**, **Scott's pi** and the related **Fleiss' kappa**, **inter-rater correlation**, **concordance correlation coefficient** and **intra-class correlation**. For established the reliability of present sports injury inventory Intera-class correlation method was used.

Intra-Class Correlation Coefficient

There are several types of this method and one of them defined as, "the proportion of variance of an observation due to between-subject variability in the true scores". he range of the intra-class correlation may be between 0.0 and 1.0. The intra-class correlation will be high when there is little variation between the scores given to each item by the raters, e.g. if all raters give the same, or similar scores to each of the items. The obtained value of Intra-class correlation was .880 which show that inventory was significant reliable.

For detail regarding developed inventory please refer appendix

III.4 Administration of Injury Report Inventory

1. For each category of sample, by and large the research scholar has approached to them individually.

2. After ensuring the availability of time, the purpose of the study has been explained to the respondents.
3. Once they understood and agreed to responses and participated in the study, consent has been taken.
4. Thereafter required inventory has been distributed to the subjects and requested to read once carefully without giving any response.
5. Doubt or confusion of respondents were finally cleared or explained.
6. In case of language, the research scholar read out and explained the meaning of questions, and noted down the required response.
7. After ensuring that they have understood and concerned individual was prepared for responding, the required inventory was got filled up by the respondents.

III.5 Data Collection

The researcher personally visited the desired destinations to fulfillment their research work of sports injuries. The data has been collected from the All India Universities Competitions held at different campuses of Indian Universities. Each injury episode during training or match-play was outlined in a detailed injury report form that was completed by experts of sports medicines. The injury reports form comprise a questionnaire of the injury specific including, injury, body part associated, time lost due to injury (for severity purpose), injury classification, injury type, playing surface and reason of injury with match-play events associated with injuries. All injuries assessed after the confirmation of a physiotherapist whom were presented at the time of competition to ensure the accuracy of details when completing injury record documentation.

The description of the All India-University competitions where the data had been collected given below:

Table III-2 Description of Events

Game	Date	Venue
Cricket	22-30 Nov 2017	M D U, Rohtak

Baseball	14-18 Nov 2017	M D U Rohtak
Kabaddi	19-23 Nov 2017	M. D. U, Rohtak
Basketball	26-30 Dec 2017	JMI. N. Delhi
Hockey	1st Oct 2017	NHIS, Delhi
Football	22-30 Nov 2017	D.B. University
Wrestling	3-5 Nov 2017	M D U, Rohtak
Wt. Lifting	4-6 Nov 2017	Chandigarh University, Mohali
Badminton	1-4 Dec 2017	M D U, Rohtak
Boxing	1-4 Feb 2018	Chandigarh
Gymnastic	15-18 Jan	KUK, Kurukshetra
Judo	22-24 Feb 2018	Chandigarh

III.6 Statistical Techniques Used for Analysis of the Data

The purpose of the present study was to compare the common sports injuries between team and individual sports competitions. For accomplish the study following statistical tools were used to analysis the raw data:

- Percentage
- Injury ranking
- Normal Curve Distribution
- Chi-square

Percentage

In its simplest form, percent mean per hundred. To definite a number between zero and one, percentage formula is used. It is defines as a number represented as a fraction of 100. Symbolized by the symbol = %, it is majorly used to compare and finding out ratios. The Percentage Formula is given as,

Percentage=————

Normal Curve Distribution

First step:

- Mean: $\frac{\Sigma x}{N}$

- Standard Deviation: $\sqrt{\frac{\Sigma d^2}{N}}$

Second step

- A normal curve covers ±3σ
- : Total distance = 6σ
- To grade the injury severity into 5 categories in the normal curve within 6σ limit.
- Each grade curve = $\frac{6\sigma}{5}$ = 1.2σ

Third Step:

Thus to find out the area covered by each grade in the normal curve i.e. ±3σ. Standard score formula $\{z = \frac{x-M}{\sigma}\}$ is employed to find out the range of each point to categorize the grade.

- Critical: x=3×SD+Mean
- Severe: x= 1.8×SD+Mean
- Serious: x=6×SD+Mean
- Moderate: x= -.6×SD+Mean
- Minor : x=-1.8×SD+Mean

Thus to calculate the lowest range, we have to calculate the lower limit here,

- X= -3×SD+Mean

Fourth step:

To get the range of all desired grade the upper limit of corresponding scale will be subtracted from the upper limit of next below.

Non Parametric Statistics

Non-parametric statistics makes weaker and fewer assumptions about the characteristic of the population distribution. Depend only sparingly on the latter, do not involve the population parameters, and can be applied irrespectively or sample size and population distribution or even for nomination or ordinal variables.

Where use:

- Non-parametric statistics can be applied to the data involving nominal or ordinal variables and too small sample or samples drawn from non-normally distributed population.
- Most non-parametric test that used for testing experimental hypothesis and for analyzing the observed frequencies and variance, are less complicated and speedier in calculation than parametric ones.
- Non-parametric tests are less appropriate than parametric tests for ratio and interval variables.
- Less powerful than that of parametric statistics.

Chi-square (x^2)

a non-parametric test is conventionally called the chi square test because the statistics computed for it has a x^2 sampling distribution. It is a generalized expression between a theoretical and actual distribution, i.e. an actual response as related to an expected responses. It can be used with either parametric or non-parametric data.

$$X^2 = \frac{\left(O_i^I - E_i\right)^2}{E_i}$$

Where,

O_i = frequency of occurrence or observed.

E_i = frequency of occurrence as indicated by some hypothesis or expected.

Chi-square Test of Independence.

x^2 test are used to find whether there is a significant association between two variables in a sample or the two variables are independent or each other.

Chapter – IV

ANALYSIS OF THE DATA AND RESULTS OF THE STUDY

Chapter-IV

ANALYSIS OF THE DATA AND RESULT OF THE STUDY

Overview

Chapter-IV

ANALYSIS OF THE DATA & RESULTS OF THE STUDY

IV. **Results of the Study**

The purpose of this study was to compare the common sports injuries between the team game and individual sports competition. For accomplish the study a total 300 players were selected as sample through random sample technique. Out of the total sample 150 players were from team games and 150 players were from individual sports competition.

To assess the common sports injuries a well-structured injury report inventory (IRV) (see appendix) was used. The injury report inventory consists of the following variables:

- Common sports injuries
- Body parts associated with injuries
- Injury severity (based on time lost in days from practice)
- Injury occurred during Match/Training
- Injury classification
- Ground surfaces

There was a separate section in the injury report form to appraise the possible reasons of injuries which was further divided into two sections given below:

1. Intrinsic reason
2. Extrinsic reason

This chapter summarizes the obtained results with the help of pre-defined methodology in 3rd chapter of this thesis. Without the statistical techniques we are not able to understand our raw data. Research data is a useless phenomenon until performed statistical computations.

As per the nature of this study and the injury report form used to assess the common sports injuries which was almost an open ended questionnaire. So this study based on non-parametric assumptions. Chi-square a non-parametric measure of statistics was used to compare the obtained responses between team and individual sports of sports injuries. Percentage and frequency distribution was used to explain injury statements. Injury rate per 100 athletes was also used to assess the injury rate within selected and individual sports.

IV.1 Descriptive Statistics

Table IV-1 Case summaries

Game Type		Age (Years)	Height (cm)	Weight (kg)	Experience (Years)	Training Hours
Team game	N	150	150	150	150	150
	Mean	20.59	173.2954	68.49	6.34	4.15
	SEM	.181	.59076	.868	.228	.088
	SD	2.236	7.28340	10.698	2.815	1.086
	Minimum	17	152.40	34	1	2
	Maximum	29	198.12	100	20	6
	% of Total N	50%	50%	50%	50%	50%
	Skewness	1.050	.208	.366	.898	.149
	Kurtosis	1.758	1.083	.999	2.364	-.199
Individual Game	N	150	150	150	150	150
	Mean	20.04	173.5212	72.29	4.83	4.34
	SEM	.256	.67511	1.270	.285	.075
	SD	3.119	8.21303	15.450	3.467	.916
	Minimum	15	144.78	42	1	2
	Maximum	33	195.58	130	20	8
	% of Total N	50%	50%	50%	50%	50%
	Skewness	1.574	-.235	.681	1.434	.173
	Kurtosis	3.565	1.093	.620	2.785	1.645
Total	N	300	300	300	300	300
	Mean	20.32	173.4068	70.36	5.60	4.24
	SEM	.157	.44709	.772	.187	.058
	SD	2.717	7.74376	13.371	3.238	1.009
	Minimum	15	144.78	34	1	2
	Maximum	33	198.12	130	20	8
	% of Total N	100.0%	100.0%	100.0%	100.0%	100.0%
	Skewness	1.358	-.045	.756	1.018	.107
	Kurtosis	3.300	1.096	1.323	1.978	.462

The table 4.1 explores the case summaries of the selected sample further divided into team and individual sports competitions. The descriptive statistics for the present study was analyzed in the terms of mean, standard error mean, standard deviation, minimum, maximum, percent of total No. of subject, skewness and kurtosis. Age, height, weight, experience and training hours were the variables which characteristics were carried out with the help of descriptive statistics. The mean score for the team game in their age was 20.59, standard error mean was 0.181, standard deviation was 2.236, minimum and maximum magnitude of age was ranged from 17±29 years, percentage of total N (No. of respondents) in age was 50.7%, skewness and kurtosis were 1.050±1.758. The mean score of height was 173.29 standard error of mean was 0.590, standard deviation was 7.283 and range of minimum and maximum values of height were 152.40±198.12, percentage of total no. of respondents in height were 50% (150) and skewness and kurtosis for height were .208±1.08 respectively. Mean score of third variable weight were 68.49, standard error mean were 0.868, standard deviation were 10.698, minimum and maximum values for weight were 34±100 kg, percentage of total N were same 50.7% and skewness and kurtosis for weight were 0.366±0.999. The summaries of experience for the team game respondents were as follow; mean score of experience were 6.34 years, standard error mean was 0.228, standard deviation was 2.815, minimum and maximum experience in team game was 1±20 years, percentage of total N was 50.7% and skewness and kurtosis were 0.898±2.634. Training hours denotes the total practicing hours in one day. The mean of training hours was 4.15 hours, standard error mean was 0.088, standard deviation was 1.086, minimum and maximum values for training hours were 2±6, percentage of total N (no. of respondents) was 50.5% (151) and skewness and kurtosis for training hours were 0.149±0.199

The mean score of **Individual game** in their age was 20.04 years, standard error mean was 0.256, standard deviation was 3.119, minimum and maximum valued of age were 15±33 years, percentage of total N (no. of respondents) in individual games were 49.3%, skewness and kurtosis were 1.574±3.565, the average height in individual games was 173.52, standard error mean was 0.675, standard deviation was 8.21, minimum and maximum values for height in individual games were 144.78±195.58, percentage of total N was 49.3% , skewness and kurtosis for height were -0.235±1.093

respectively. The characteristics of weight in individual games were as follow. The mean score of weight is 72.29 kg, standard error mean is 1.270, standard deviation is 15.450 minimum and maximum weight is 42±130, percentage of total N is 49.3%, skewness and kurtosis is 0.681±0.620. The mean score of experience in individual games are 4.83 years, standard error mean of experience is 0.285, standard deviation is 3.467, minimum and maximum values are ranged from1±20 years, percentage of total N is 50%, skewness and kurtosis for experience is 1.434±2.785 respectively. Mean score of training hours is 4.34, standard error mean is 0.075, standard deviation is 0.916, minimum and maximum values are 2±8 years, percentage of total N is 49.5%, skewness and kurtosis are 0.173±1.645.

Observation in table **4.1** also reveals the characteristics of **total sample (N=300)** and mean score of **age** of total sample is 20.32, standard error mean is 0.157, standard deviation is 2.717, minimum and maximum values for age of total sample are15±33, percentage of total N is 100%, skewness and kurtosis are 1.358±3.300 respectively. The mean score of **height** of total sample is 173.40 cm, standard error mean is 0.447, standard deviation is 7.74, minimum and maximum score of height are ranged from 144.78 cm (minimum height) to 198.12 cm (maximum height). Percentage of total N is 100%, skewness and kurtosis are -0.045±1.096. The average **weight** is 70.36 kg found in total sample, standard error mean is 0.772, standard deviation is 13.371, minimum and maximum values are 34±130 kg, percentage of total N 100%, skewness and kurtosis are 0.756±1.323. The mean for **experience** in total sample is 5.60, standard error mean is 0.187, standard deviation is 3.23, minimum and maximum values are 1±20 years, percentage of total N is 100%, skewness and kurtosis are 1.018±1.978. Score of training hours in total sample is 4.24 hours, standard error mean is 0.058, standard deviation is1.009, minimum and maximum training hours are 2±8 hours, percentage of total N is 100% (300), skewness and kurtosis are 0.107±0.462.

Figure IV-1 Graphical Presentation of Mean and Standard Deviation of Team and Individual Score in Their Age, Height, Weight, Experience and Training Hours

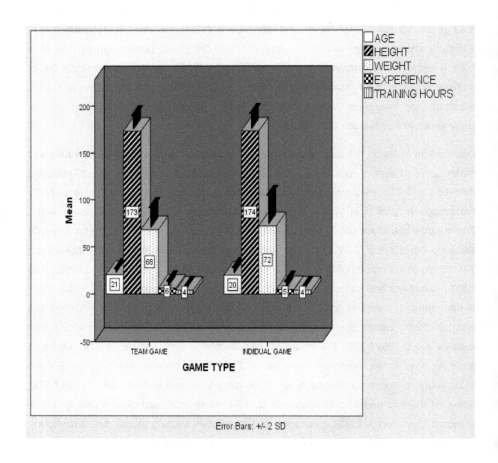

Error Bars: +/- 2 SD

Table IV-2 Descriptive Statistics Cricket

	Age (Years)	Height (cm)	Weight (kg)	Experience (Years)	Training Hours
N	25	25	25	25	25
Mean	20.88	172.0085	68.12	6.50	5.38
Std. Error of Mean	.512	1.14768	1.862	.572	.167
Std. Deviation	2.613	5.85205	9.497	2.915	.852
Minimum	18	160.02	54	2	4
Maximum	26	185.42	90	11	6
% of Total N	8.33%	8.33%	8.33%	8.33%	8.33%
Skewness	.588	.224	.705	.089	-.870

The descriptive statistics of cricket players is being presented in table 4.2 it was analyzed that the mean score of **age** is 20.88 years, standard error of mean is 0.512, standard deviation is 2.613, minimum and maximum values are 18±26 years, percentage of total N is 8.7% and skewness is 0.588.

The mean score of **height** is 172.008 cm, standard error of mean is 1.147, standard deviation is 5.85, minimum and maximum values are 160.02±185.42 cm , percentage of total N is 8.7% and skewness is 0.224.

The mean score of **weight** is 68.12 kg, standard error mean is 1.862, standard deveiation is 9.49, minimum and maximum values are 54±90, percentage of total N is 8.7% and skewness is 0.705.

The mean score of **experience** is 6.50 years, standard error mean is 0.572, standard deviation is 2.91, minimum and maximum values are 2±11 years and skewnes is 0.089 respectively.

The mean score of training hours is 5.38 hours, standard error mean is 0.167, standard deviation is 0.852, minimum and maximum values are 4±6, percentage of total N is 8.7%, and skewness is -0.870.

Table IV-3 Descriptive Statistics Baseball

	Age (Years)	Height (cm)	Weight (kg)	Experience (Years)	Training Hours
N	25	25	25	25	25
Mean	20.55	172.0917	66.45	5.86	3.72
Std. Error of Mean	.353	1.29548	2.557	.486	.130
Std. Deviation	1.901	6.97639	13.767	2.615	.702
Minimum	18	154.00	34	2	2
Maximum	24	182.00	100	13	5
% of Total N	8.33%	8.33%	8.33%	8.33%	8.33%
Skewness	.333	-.775	.226	.844	-1.551

The descriptive statistics of Baseball players is being presented in table 4.3 it was analyzed that the mean score of **age** is 20.55 years, standard error of mean is 0.353, standard deviation is 1.901, minimum and maximum values are 18±24 years, percentage of total N is 9.7% and skewness is 0.333

The mean score of **height** is 172.09 cm, standard error of mean is 1.29, standard deviation is 6.97, minimum and maximum values are 154±182 cm , percentage of total N is 9.7% and skewness is -0.775.

The mean score of **weight** is 66.45 kg, standard error mean is 2.55, standard deveiation is 13.67, minimum and maximum values are 34±100, percentage of total N is 9.7% and skewness is 0.226.

The mean score of **experience** is 5.86 years, standard error mean is 0.486, standard deviation is 2.615, minimum and maximum values are 2±13 years and skewnes is 0.844 respectively.

The mean score of **training hours** is 3.72 hours, standard error mean is 0.130, standard deviation is 0.702, minimum and maximum values are 2±5, percentage of total N is 8.33%, and skewness is -1.55.

Table IV-4 Descriptive Statistics Kabaddi

	Age (Years)	Height (cm)	Weight (kg)	Experience (Years)	Training Hours
N	25	25	25	25	25
Mean	20.91	170.1270	72.57	6.83	4.00
Std. Error of Mean	.453	1.36441	1.531	.498	.000
Std. Deviation	2.172	6.54346	7.341	2.387	.000
Minimum	18	152.40	55	3	4
Maximum	27	180.34	91	10	4
% of Total N	8.33%	8.33%	8.33%	8.33%	8.33%
Skewness	.850	-.938	.297	.049	.

The descriptive statistics of Kabaddi players is being presented in table 4.4 it was analyzed that the mean score of **age** is 20.91 years, standard error of mean is 0.453, standard deviation is 2.172, minimum and maximum values are 18±27 years, percentage of total N is 7.7% and skewness is 0.850.

The mean score of **height** is 170.12 cm, standard error of mean is 1.36, standard deviation is 6.54, minimum and maximum values are 152.40±180.34 cm , percentage of total N is 7.7% and skewness is -0.938.

The mean score of **weight** is 72.57 kg, standard error mean is 1.531, standard deveiation is 7.341, minimum and maximum values are 55±91, percentage of total N is 7.7% and skewness is 0.297.

The mean score of **experience** is 6.83, standard error mean is 0.498, standard deviation is 2.38, minimum and maximum values are 3±10 years and skewnes is 0.049 respectively.

The mean score of **training hours** is 4 hours, standard error mean is 0.00, standard deviation is 0.00, minimum and maximum values are 4±4, percentage of total N is 8.33%, and skewness is(cannot computed).

Table IV-5 Descriptive Statistics Basketball

	Age (Years)	Height (cm)	Weight (kg)	Experience (Years)	Training Hours
N	25	25	25	25	25
Mean	21.62	173.3676	71.67	6.81	3.90
Std. Error of Mean	.475	1.74799	3.071	.847	.194
Std. Deviation	2.179	8.01029	14.072	3.881	.889
Minimum	18	152.40	49	2	2
Maximum	29	182.88	97	20	5
% of Total N	8.33%	8.33%	8.33%	8.33%	8.33%
Skewness	1.793	-1.057	.303	2.161	-.744

The descriptive statistics of Basketball players is being presented in table 4.5 it was analyzed that the mean score of **age** is 21.62 years, standard error of mean is 0.547, standard deviation is 2.179, minimum and maximum values are 18±29 years, percentage of total N is .0% and skewness is 1.793.

The mean score of **height** is 173.36 cm, standard error of mean is 1.74, standard deviation is 8.01, minimum and maximum values are 152.40±182.88 cm , percentage of total N is 7.0% and skewness is -1.057.

The mean score of **weight** is 71.67 kg, standard error mean is 3.071, standard deveiation is 14.072, minimum and maximum values are 49±97, percentage of total N is 7% and skewness is 0.303.

The mean score of **experience** is 6.81 years, standard error mean is 0.847, standard deviation is 3.881, minimum and maximum values are 2±20 years and skewnes is 2.161 respectively.

The mean score of training hours is 3.90 hours, standard error mean is 0.194, standard deviation is 0.889, minimum and maximum values are 2±5, percentage of total N is 8.33%, and skewness is -0.744.

Table IV-6 Descriptive Statistics Hockey

	Age	Height	Weight	Experience	Training
	(Years)	(cm)	(kg)	(Years)	Hours
N	25	25	25	25	25
Mean	21.10	172.6219	67.71	7.86	4.81
Std. Error of Mean	.547	1.52186	2.224	.464	.214
Std. Deviation	2.508	6.97403	10.194	2.128	.981
Minimum	18	154.00	49	3	3
Maximum	29	182.00	85	12	6
% of Total N	8.33%	8.33%	8.33%	8.33%	8.33%
Skewness	1.794	-1.050	.069	-.482	.067

The descriptive statistics of Hockey players is being presented in table 4.6 it was analyzed that the mean score of **age** is 21.10 years, standard error of mean is 0.547, standard deviation is 2.50, minimum and maximum values are 18±29 years, percentage of total N is 7.0% and skewness is 1.794.

The mean score of **height** is 172.62 cm, standard error of mean is 1.521, standard deviation is 6.97, minimum and maximum values are 154.±182 cm , percentage of total N is 7.0% and skewness is -1.050.

The mean score of **weight** is 67.71 kg, standard error mean is 2.22, standard deveiation is 10.194, minimum and maximum values are 49±85, percentage of total N is 7.0% and skewness is 0.069.

The mean score of **experience** is 7.860 years, standard error mean is 0.464, standard deviation is 2.12, minimum and maximum values are 3±12 years and skewnes is -0.482 respectively.

The mean score of **training hours** is 4.81 hours, standard error mean is 214, standard deviation is 0.981, minimum and maximum values are 3±6, percentage of total N is 8.33%, and skewness is 0.067.

Table IV-7 Descriptive Statistics Football

	Age (Years)	Height (cm)	Weight (kg)	Experience (Years)	Training Hours
N	25	25	25	25	25
Mean	19.16	174.2788	71.13	5.00	3.34
Std. Error of Mean	.246	1.65905	2.906	.391	.183
Std. Deviation	1.394	9.38502	16.441	2.214	1.035
Minimum	17	152.40	46	1	2
Maximum	22	198.12	122	10	6
% of Total N	8.33%	8.33%	8.33%	8.33%	8.33%
Skewness	.390	.277	1.136	.304	.913

The descriptive statistics of Football players is being presented in table 4.7 it was analyzed that the mean score of **age** is 19.16 years, standard error of mean is 0.246, standard deviation is 1.394, minimum and maximum values are 17±22 years, percentage of total N is 10.7% and skewness is 1.794.

The mean score of **height** is 174.27 cm, standard error of mean is 1.659, standard deviation is 9.38, minimum and maximum values are 152.40±198.12 cm , percentage of total N is 10.7% and skewness is 0.277.

The mean score of **weight** is 71.13 kg, standard error mean is 2.90, standard deviation is 16.44, minimum and maximum values are 46±122, percentage of total N is 10.7% and skewness is 1.136.

The mean score of **experience** is 5.00 years, standard error mean is 0.391, standard deviation is 2.214, minimum and maximum values are 1±10 years and skewness is 0.304 respectively.

The mean score **of training hours** is 3.34 hours, standard error mean is 0.183, standard deviation is 1.035, minimum and maximum values are 2±6, percentage of total N is 8.33%, and skewness is 0.913.

Table IV-8 Descriptive Statistics Wrestling

	Age (Years)	Height (cm)	Weight (kg)	Experience (Years)	Training Hours
N	25	25	25	25	25
Mean	20.19	175.2031	81.54	5.15	4.15
Std. Error of Mean	.372	2.13991	3.234	.483	.154
Std. Deviation	1.898	10.91147	16.491	2.461	.784
Minimum	17	144.78	59	2	2
Maximum	27	193.04	130	10	5
% of Total N	8.33%	8.33%	8.33%	8.33%	8.33%
Skewness	1.717	-.457	.826	.471	-.825

The descriptive statistics of wrestling players is being presented in table 4.8 it was analyzed that the mean score of **age** is 20.19 years, standard error of mean is 0.372, standard deviation is 1.898, minimum and maximum values are 17±27 years, percentage of total N is 8.7% and skewness is 1.717.

The mean score of **height** is 175.20 cm, standard error of mean is 2.13, standard deviation is 10.91, minimum and maximum values are 144.78±193.04 cm, percentage of total N is 8.7% and skewness is -0.457.

The mean score of **weight** is 81.54 kg, standard error mean is 3.23, standard deviation is 16.49, minimum and maximum values are 59±130, percentage of total N is 8.7% and skewness is 0.826.

The mean score of **experience** is 5.15 years, standard error mean is 0.483, standard deviation is 2.46, minimum and maximum values are 2±10 years and skewnes is 0.471 respectively.

The mean score of training hours is 4.15 hours, standard error mean is 0.154, standard deviation is 0.784, minimum and maximum values are 2±5, percentage of total N is 8.33%, and skewness is -0.825.

Table IV-9 Descriptive Statistics Weight Lifting

	Age (Years)	Height (cm)	Weight (kg)	Experience (Years)	Training Hours
N	25	25	25	25	25
Mean	21.50	175.4780	90.45	3.90	3.95
Std. Error of Mean	.635	1.01349	2.292	.661	.114
Std. Deviation	2.838	4.53246	10.252	2.954	.510
Minimum	18	170.18	79	1	3
Maximum	28	182.88	122	10	5
% of Total N	8.33%	8.33%	8.33%	8.33%	8.33%
Skewness	.660	.157	1.713	.871	-.112

The descriptive statistics of Weight Lifters is being presented in table 4.9 it was analyzed that the mean score of **age** is 21.50 years, standard error of mean is 0.635, standard deviation is 2.838, minimum and maximum values are 18±28 years, percentage of total N is 6.7% and skewness is 0.660.

The mean score of **height** is 175.47 cm, standard error of mean is 1.01, standard deviation is 4.53, minimum and maximum values are 170.18±182.88 cm , percentage of total N is 6.7% and skewness is 0.157.

The mean score of **weight** is 90.45 kg, standard error mean is 2.292, standard deviation is 10.252, minimum and maximum values are 79±122, percentage of total N is 6.7% and skewness is 1.713.

The mean score of **experience** is 3.90 years, standard error mean is 0.661, standard deviation is 2.95, minimum and maximum values are 1±10 years and skewnes is 0.871 respectively.

The mean score of **training hours** is 3.95 hours, standard error mean is 0.114, standard deviation is 0.510, minimum and maximum values are 3±5, percentage of total N is 8.33%, and skewness is -0.112.

Table IV-10 Descriptive Statistics Badminton

	Age (Years)	Height (cm)	Weight (kg)	Experience (Years)	Training Hours
N	25	25	25	25	25
Mean	20.47	172.4212	64.35	4.41	4.76
Std. Error of Mean	.333	2.30380	2.660	.364	.161
Std. Deviation	1.375	9.49882	10.966	1.502	.664
Minimum	19	152.40	49	2	3
Maximum	24	182.88	87	7	6
% of Total N	8.33%	8.33%	8.33%	8.33%	8.33%
Skewness	1.296	-1.050	.697	.192	-1.159

The descriptive statistics of Badminton players is being presented in table 4.10 and it was analyzed that the mean score of **age** is 20.47 years, standard error of mean is 0.333, standard deviation is 1.375, minimum and maximum values are 19±24 years, percentage of total N is 5.7% and skewness is 1.296.

The mean score of **height** is 172.42 cm, standard error of mean is 2.30, standard deviation is 9.49, minimum and maximum values are 152.40±182.88 cm , percentage of total N is 5.7% and skewness is -1.050.

The mean score of **weight** is 64.35 kg, standard error mean is 2.66, standard deviation is 10.96, minimum and maximum values are 49±87, percentage of total N is 5.7% and skewness is 0.697.

The mean score of **experience** is 4.41 years, standard error mean is 0.364, standard deviation is 1.502, minimum and maximum values are 2±7 years and skewnes is 0.192 respectively.

The mean score of training hours is 4.76 hours, standard error mean is 0.161, standard deviation is 0.664, minimum and maximum values are 3±6, percentage of total N is 5.7%, and skewness is -1.159.

Table IV-11 Descriptive statistics Boxing

	Age (Years)	Height (cm)	Weight (kg)	Experience (Years)	Training Hours
N	25	25	25	25	25
Mean	17.50	174.8655	65.14	1.86	4.86
Std. Error of Mean	.613	1.51485	2.160	.190	.075
Std. Deviation	2.874	7.10526	10.129	.889	.351
Minimum	15	165.10	51	1	4
Maximum	28	190.54	86	4	5
% of Total N	8.33%	8.33%	8.33%	8.33%	8.33%
Skewness	2.607	.657	.548	.734	-2.278

The descriptive statistics of Boxers are being presented in table 4.11 it was analyzed that the mean score of **age** is 17.50 years, standard error of mean is 0.613, standard deviation is 2.874, minimum and maximum values are 15±28 years, percentage of total N is 7.3% and skewness is 2.607.

The mean score of **height** is 174.86 cm, standard error of mean is 1.514, standard deviation is 7.105, minimum and maximum values are 165.10±190.54 cm, percentage of total N is 7.3% and skewness is 0.657.

The mean score of **weight** is 65.14 kg, standard error mean is 2.160, standard deviation is 10.129, minimum and maximum values are 51±86, percentage of total N is 7.3% and skewness is 0.548.

The mean score of **experience** is 1.86 years, standard error mean is 0.190, standard deviation is 0.889, minimum and maximum values are 1±4 years and skewness is 0.734 respectively.

The mean score of training hours is 4.86 hours, standard error mean is 0.075, standard deviation is 0.351, minimum and maximum values are 4±5, percentage of total N is 7.3%, and skewness is -2.278.

Table IV-12 Descriptive Statistics Gymnastic

	Age (Years)	Height (cm)	Weight (kg)	Experience (Years)	Training Hours
N	25	25	25	25	25
Mean	19.57	166.6270	56.78	6.74	4.26
Std. Error of Mean	.430	1.19864	1.595	.531	.268
Std. Deviation	2.063	5.74846	7.651	2.544	1.287
Minimum	17	149.86	42	3	3
Maximum	24	175.26	69	12	8
% of Total N	8.33%	8.33%	8.33%	8.33%	8.33%
Skewness	1.123	-.806	.095	.755	1.287

The descriptive statistics of Gymnasts is being presented in table 4.12 it was analyzed that the mean score of **age** is 19.57 years, standard error of mean is 0.430, standard deviation is 2.063, minimum and maximum values are 17±24 years, percentage of total N is 7.7% and skewness is 1.123.

The mean score of **height** is 166.62 cm, standard error of mean is 1.198, standard deviation is 5.748, minimum and maximum values are 149.86±175.26 cm, percentage of total N is 7.7% and skewness is -0.806.

The mean score of **weight** is 56.78 kg, standard error mean is 1.595, standard deviation is 7.65, minimum and maximum values are 42±69, percentage of total N is 7.7% and skewness is 0.095.

The mean score of **experience** is 6.74 years, standard error mean is 0.531, standard deviation is 2.54, minimum and maximum values are 3±12 years and skewness is 0.755 respectively.

The mean score of **training hours** is 4.26 hours, standard error mean is 0.268, standard deviation is 1.287, minimum and maximum values are 3±8, percentage of total N is 87.7%, and skewness is 1.287.

Table IV-13 Descriptive Statistics Judo

	Age (Years)	Height (cm)	Weight (kg)	Experience (Years)	Training Hours
N	25	25	25	25	25
Mean	22.00	174.8000	76.87	8.94	4.44
Std. Error of Mean	1.208	1.51352	2.646	1.236	.241
Std. Deviation	4.830	6.05407	10.582	4.946	.964
Minimum	18	165.10	60	2	2
Maximum	33	183.00	96	20	6
% of Total N	8.33%	8.33%	8.33%	8.33%	8.33%
Skewness	1.334	-.234	.174	.953	-.564

The descriptive statistics of Judokas is being presented in table 4.14 and it was analyzed that the mean score of **age** is 22 years, standard error of mean is 1.208, standard deviation is 4.830, minimum and maximum values are 18±33 years, percentage of total N is 5.3% and skewness is 1.334.

The mean score of **height** is 174.80 cm, standard error of mean is 1.513, standard deviation is 6.054, minimum and maximum values are 165.10±183.00 cm, percentage of total N is 5.3% and skewness is -0.234.

The mean score of **weight** is 76.87 kg, standard error mean is 2.646, standard deviation is 10.582, minimum and maximum values are 60±96, percentage of total N is 5.3% and skewness is 0.174.

The mean score of **experience** is 8.94 years, standard error mean is 1.236, standard deviation is 4.946, minimum and maximum values are 2±20 years and skewness is 0.953 respectively.

The mean score of **training hours** is 4.44 hours, standard error mean is 0.241, standard deviation is 0.964, minimum and maximum values are 2±6, percentage of total N is 5.3%, and skewness is -0.564.

Figure IV-2   Graphical Representation of Mean Score of Age of Selected Games

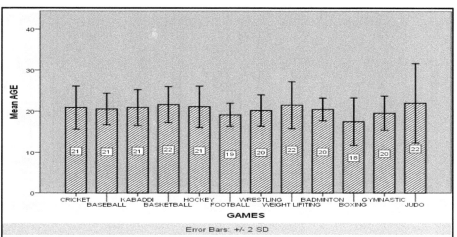

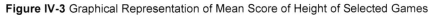

Figure IV-3 Graphical Representation of Mean Score of Height of Selected Games

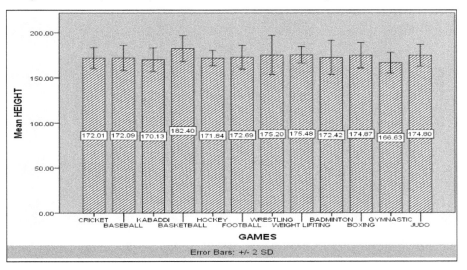

Figure IV-4 Graphical Representation of Mean Score of Weight of Selected Games

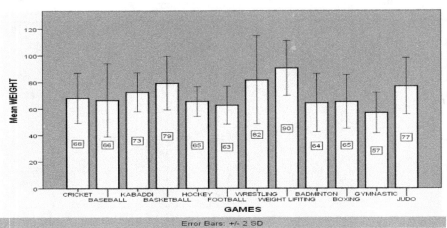

Figure IV-5 Graphical Representation of Mean Score of Experience of Selected Games

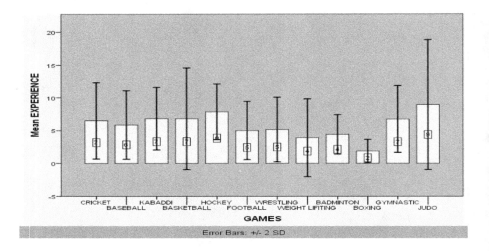

Figure IV-6 Graphical Representation of Mean Score of Training Hours of Selected Games

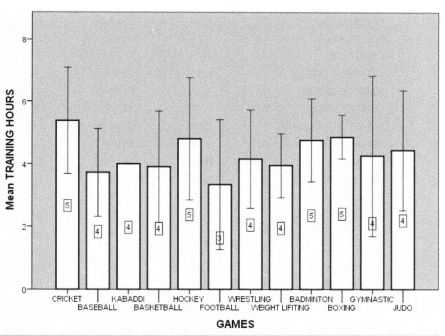

IV.2 Distribution of Common Sports Injuries

Table IV-14 Frequencies, Percentage and Rate of Common Injuries in Team Games

		Responses		Percent of	Injury
		N	Percent	cases	Ranking
Injuries	ABRASION	83	15.6%	55.7%	1
	BLISTERS	29	5.5%	19.5%	9
	CONTUSION	56	10.5%	37.6%	4
	INCISION	26	4.9%	17.4%	10
	LACERATION	23	4.3%	15.4%	11
	DISLOCATION	17	3.2%	11.4%	12
	FRACTURE	41	7.7%	27.5%	5
	LIGAMENT BREAK	29	5.5%	19.5%	9
	MUSCLE CRAMP	34	6.4%	22.8%	7
	MUSCLE PULL	57	10.7%	38.3%	3
	PUNCTURE WOUND	3	0.6%	2.0%	19
	SPRAIN	67	12.6%	45.0%	2
	STRAIN	35	6.6%	23.5%	6
	TENDINITIES	5	0.9%	3.4%	16
	CONCUSSION	4	0.8%	2.7%	17
	MENISCUS TEAR	6	1.1%	4.0%	14
	TENNIS ELBOW	5	0.9%	3.4%	16
	BACK PAIN	3	0.6%	2.0%	19
	MUSCLE TEAR	2	0.4%	1.3%	20
	ROTATOR CUFF	7	1.3%	4.7%	13
Total		532	100.0%	357.0%	

a. Dichotomy group tabulated at value 1.
b. Percentage of Injury cases.
c. Injury Ranking (1st rank denote highest score) (based on injury rate)
d. Ranks are in descending order

The table 4.15 shows frequencies, percentage and rate of injuries per 100 athletes. It's observed that in team games a total 532 injuries were recorded. Out of total, the frequency of **abrasion** is 83, percentage distribution is 15.6% and injury rate is 55.7%, frequency of **blisters** is 29 with percentage of 5.5% and injury rate is 19.5%. Frequency of **contusion** is 56 which make 10.5% and injury rate is 37.6%. Frequency of **incision** is 26, percentage distribution is 4.9% and injury rate is 17.4%. Frequency of **laceration** is 23, percentage distribution is 4.3% and rate of injury/100 athletes is 15.4%. Frequency of **dislocation** in team games are 17 with a percentage of 3.2% and injury rate is 11.4%. Frequency of **fracture** is 41, percentage distribution is 7.7% and injury rate is 27.5% respectively. Frequency of **Ligament Break** is 29, percentage distribution is 5.5% and injury rate is 19.5%. Frequency of muscle cramp is 34, percentage distribution is 6.4% and injury rate is 22.8%. Frequency of **muscle pull** is 57, percentage distribution is 10.7 and injury rate is 38.3% per hundred athletes. Frequency of **puncture wound** is 3, distribution of percentage is 0.6% and injury rate is 2%. Frequency of **Sprain** in team games are 67, percentage distribution is 12.6% and injury rate of sprain in team games are 45% respectively. Frequency of **strain** is 35, percentage distribution is 6.6% and injury rate is 23.5%. Frequency of tendinitis in team games are 5, percentage distribution is 0.9% and injury rate is 3.4%. Frequency of **concussion** is 4, percentage distribution is 0.8% and injury rate is 2.7%. In team games 6 **meniscuses tear** were recorded which consist 1.1% and injury rate of 4%. The frequency of Tennis Elbow is 5, percentage distribution is 0.9% and injury rate is 3.4%. Frequency of **Back Pain** is 3, percentage is 0.6% and injury rate is 2%. Frequency of **Muscle Tear** is 2, percentage distribution is 0.4% and injury rate is 1.3%. 7 injuries of **Rotator Cuff** were recorded in team games, percentage distribution of following injury is 1.3% and injury rate is 4.7% respectively.

As per ranking of injuries in team games 1st rank goes to injury Abrasion, second highest prone injury is Sprain which lead by muscle pull. The lowest rank (20) goes to Muscle Tear which recorded only 2 muscle tear frequencies in team game. (See the bar graph no. 4.7)

Figure IV-7 Frequencies distribution of Common Injuries in Team Games

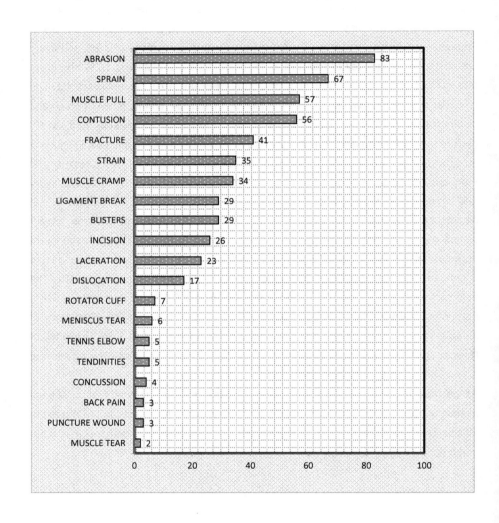

Table IV-15 Frequencies, Percentage and Rate of Common Injuries in Individual Games

		Responses		Percent of	Injury Ranking
		N	**Percent**	**cases**	
injuries	ABRASION	33	9.1%	22.4%	6
	BLISTERS	23	6.3%	15.6%	9
	CONTUSION	45	12.4%	30.6%	2
	INCISION	14	3.8%	9.5%	11
	LACRATION	7	1.9%	4.8%	12
	DISLOCATION	25	6.9%	17.0%	7
	FRACTURE	36	9.9%	24.5%	4
	LIGAMENT BREAK	23	6.3%	15.6%	9
	MUSCLE CRAMP	33	9.1%	22.4%	6
	MUSCLE PULL	50	13.7%	34.0%	1
	SPRAIN	36	9.9%	24.5%	4
	STRAIN	22	6.0%	15.0%	10
	TENDINITIES	1	0.3%	0.7%	18
	MINUSCUS TEAR	2	0.5%	1.4%	17
	TENNIS ELBOW	3	0.8%	2.0%	15
	BACK PAIN	5	1.4%	3.4%	13
	SHIN PAIN	3	0.8%	2.0%	15
	ROTATOR CUFF	3	0.8%	2.0%	15
Total		**364**	**100.0%**	**247.6%**	

a. Dichotomy group tabulated at value 1.

b Percentage of Injury cases.

c. Injury Ranking (1st rank denote highest score) (based on injury rate)

d. Ranks are in descending order

Table no. 4.16 reveals the frequencies, percentage and rate of injuries and after analysis the table, frequencies, percentage distribution and rate of injuries of **Abrasion** is 33,9.1±22.4, for **Blisters** it is 23, 6.3±15.6, for **Contusion** it is 45, 12.4±30.6, for

Incision it is 14, 3.8±9.5, for **Laceration** it is 7, 1.9±4.8, for **Dislocation** it is 25, 6.9±17, for **Fracture** it is 36, 9.9±24.5, for **Ligament Break** it is 23, 6.3±15.6, for **Muscle Cramp** it is 33, 9.1±22.4, for **Muscle Pull** it is 50, 13.7±34, for **Sprain** 36, 9.9±24.5, for **Strain** it is 22, 6±15, for **Tendinitis** it is 1, 0.3±0.7, for **Minuscus Tear** it is 2, 0.5±1.4, for **Tennis Elbow** it is 3, 0.8±2, for **Back Pain** it is 5, 1.4±3.4, for **Shin Pain** it is 3, 0.8±2 and for **Rotator Cuff** the frequencies, percentage distribution and rate of injury is 3, 0.8±2 respectively.

As per injury ranking provided in table 4.16, the most frequent injury in Individual games in Muscle Pull which lead by Contusion. The lowest frequent injury is Tendinitis found in Individual games

Figure IV-8 Frequencies distribution of Common Injuries in Individual Games

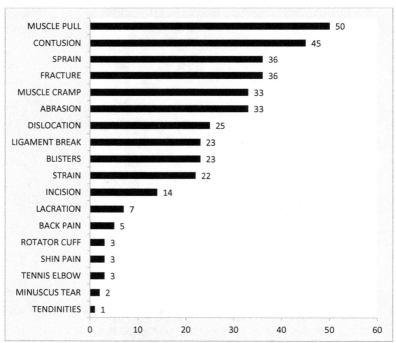

Figure IV-9 Percentage Distribution of Common Injuries between Team and Individual Sports Competition

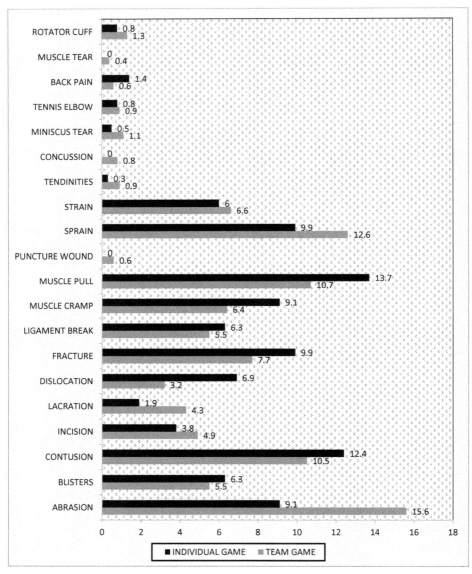

Table IV-16 **Frequencies, Percentage and Rate of Common Injuries in Cricket**

		Responses		Percent of	Injury
		N	Percent	cases	Ranking
Injuries	ABRASION	16	23.9%	61.5%	2
	BLISTERS	2	3.0%	7.7%	9
	CONTUSION	5	7.5%	19.2%	5
	INCISION	1	1.5%	3.8%	12
	LACERATION	1	1.5%	3.8%	12
	FRACTURE	5	7.5%	19.2%	5
	LIGAMENT_RUPTURE	1	1.5%	3.8%	12
	MUSCLE_CRAMP	3	4.5%	11.5%	8
	MUSCLE_PULL	17	25.4%	65.4%	1
	SPRAIN	7	10.4%	26.9%	3
	STRAIN	5	7.5%	19.2%	5
	TENDINITIES	1	1.5%	3.8%	12
	TENNIS_ELBOW	3	4.5%	11.5%	8
Total		**67**	**100.0%**	**257.7%**	

a. Dichotomy group tabulated at value 1.
b. Percentage of Injury cases
c. Injury Ranking (1st rank denote highest score) (based on injury rate)
d. Ranks are in descending order

Frequencies, percentage distribution and injury rate of common injuries of Cricketers are presented in table 4.17 and it is observed that muscle pull is highest prone injury found in Cricket with injury rate of 65.4% and got 1st rank among all injuries. Out of total injuries (67) 17 muscle pull are recorded which consist 25.4% out of 100. Second most possible injury in Cricket is Abrasion with injury rate of 61.5%. Total 16 Abrasions were recorded during data collection and percentage distribution is 23.9%. Third highest prone injury in Cricket is Sprain with IR of 26.9%. A total 7 Sprains were recorded and percentage distribution is 10.4% respectively. Incision, laceration and Tendinitis are found to be lowest injury Rate and got last common rank (12).

Figure IV-10 **Percentage Distribution of Common Injuries in Cricket**

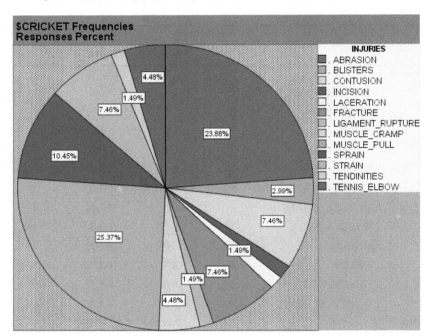

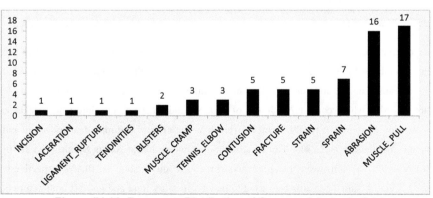

Figure IV-11 Frequency Distribution of Common Injuries in Cricket

Table IV-17 Frequencies, Percentage and Rate of Common Injuries in Baseball

		Responses		Percent of Cases	Injury Ranking
		N	Percent		
Injuries	ABRASION	11	13.6%	39.3%	2
	BLISTERS	8	9.9%	28.6%	5
	CONTUSION	9	11.1%	32.1%	4
	INCISION	1	1.2%	3.6%	16
	LACERATION	3	3.7%	10.7%	10
	DISLOCATION	2	2.5%	7.1%	13
	FRACTURE	3	3.7%	10.7%	10
	LIGAMENT RUPTURE	4	4.9%	14.3%	7
	MUSCLE CRAMP	3	3.7%	10.7%	10
	MUSCLE PULL	12	14.8%	42.9%	1
	PUNCTURE WOUND	1	1.2%	3.6%	16
	SPRAIN	6	7.4%	21.4%	6
	STRAIN	10	12.3%	35.7%	3
	TENDINITIES	1	1.2%	3.6%	16
	TENNIS ELBOW	1	1.2%	3.6%	16
	BACK PAIN	1	1.2%	3.6%	16
	MUSCLE TEAR	2	2.5%	7.1%	13
	ROTATOR CUFF	3	3.7%	10.7%	10
Total		81	100.0%	289.3%	

a. Dichotomy group tabulated at value 1.
b. Percentage of Injury cases.
c. Injury Ranking (1st rank denote highest score) (based on injury rate)
d. Ranks are in descending order

The table 4.17 explores the frequencies, percentage distribution and injury rate per 100 athletes of Baseball players. Injury ranking is also computed on the basis of injury rate. After analysis the table it observed that total 81 injuries were recorded from Baseball players. Highest frequent injury found in Baseball is muscle pull. Total 12 muscle pull were recorded during data collection and IR of muscle pull is 42.9% and percentage distribution is 14.8%. Second most frequent injury in Baseball is Abrasion with IR of 39.3% and percentage distribution of 13.6% out of hundred. Incision, Tendinitis, Puncture Wound, Tennis Elbow and Back Pain are lowest frequent injuries in Baseball and got last and common rank (16) respectively.

Figure IV-12 Percentage Distribution of Common Injuries in Baseball

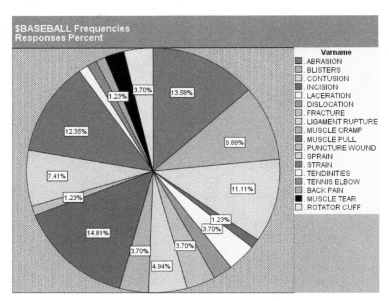

Figure IV-13 Frequency Distribution of Common injuries in Baseball

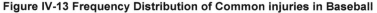

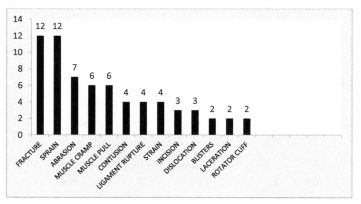

Table IV-18 Frequencies, Percentage and Rate of Common Injuries in Kabaddi

		Responses		Percent of	Injury
		N	Percent	cases	Ranking
	ABRASION	10	17.5%	43.5%	2
	CONTUSION	5	8.8%	21.7%	4
	INCISION	3	5.3%	13.0%	8
	LACERATION	3	5.3%	13.0%	8
.a Injuries	DISLOCATION	6	10.5%	26.1%	5
	FRACTURE	9	15.8%	39.1%	3
	LIGAMENT RUPTURE	3	5.3%	13.0%	8
	MUSCLE CRAMP	1	1.8%	4.3%	11
	MUSCLE PULL	3	5.3%	13.0%	8
	SPRAIN	13	22.8%	56.5%	1
	STRAIN	1	1.8%	4.3%	11
Total		57	100.0%	247.8%	

a. Dichotomy group tabulated at value 1.
b. Percentage of Injury cases
c. Injury Ranking (1st rank denote highest score) (based on injury rate)
d. Ranks are in descending order

Table 4.18 shows the frequencies distribution, percentage and injury rate of Kabaddi players. Ranks are assigned in descending order means, highest value goes 1st rank. After analysis the table it is observed that Sprain is highest frequent injury in Kabaddi. Out of total (57) injuries 13 Sprain injuries were recorded. Percentage distribution and injury rate (IR) of Sprain is 22.8±56.5 respectively. Second most frequent injury is Abrasion with IR 43.5% and a percentage of 17.5%. Third rank goes to Fracture and percentage distribution and IR of fracture is 15.8±39.1 respectively. Muscle cramp and strain are the lowest frequent injuries. Only 1 muscle cramp and strain were recorded from Kabaddi players. It should also be a considerable fact to know that fracture, ligament rupture and dislocation are has a considerable amount of injury rate in Kabaddi.

Figure IV-14 **Percentage Distribution of Common Injuries in Kabaddi**

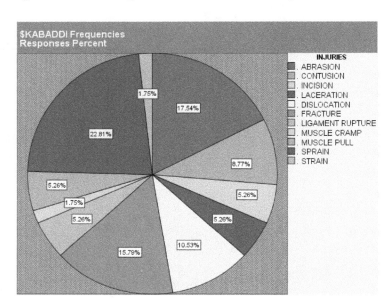

Figure IV-15 Frequency Distribution of Common Injuries in Kabaddi

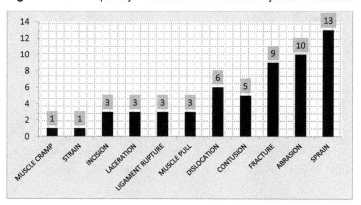

Table IV-19 Frequencies, Percentage and Rate of Common Injuries in Basketball

		Responses		Percent of	Injury
		N	Percent	Cases	Ranking
Injuries	ABRASION	7	10.4%	36.8%	3
	BLISTERS	2	3.0%	10.5%	12
	CONTUSION	4	6.0%	21.1%	7
	INCISION	3	4.5%	15.8%	10
	LACERATION	2	3.0%	10.5%	12
	DISLOCATION	3	4.5%	15.8%	10
	FRACTURE	12	17.9%	63.2%	2
	LIGAMENT RUPTURE	4	6.0%	21.1%	7
	MUSCLE CRAMP	6	9.0%	31.6%	5
	MUSCLE PULL	6	9.0%	31.6%	5
	SPRAIN	12	17.9%	63.2%	2
	STRAIN	4	6.0%	21.1%	7
	ROTATOR CUFF	2	3.0%	10.5%	12
Total		**67**	**100.0%**	**352.6%**	

a. Dichotomy group tabulated at value 1.
b. Percentage of Injury cases.
c. Injury Ranking (1st rank denote highest score) (based on injury rate)
d. Ranks are in descending order

Table 4.19 shows the dispersion of common injuries in Basketball and it is analyzed that fracture and sprain are highest possible injuries in Basketball. A total 67 injuries were recorded with the help of injury report form and out of total 12 are sprain and 12 are fracture. The injury rate of both injuries is 63.2% respectively. Second most prone injuries in Basketball are muscle cramp and muscle pull. Frequency of muscle pull is 6, percentage distribution is 9% and injury rate is 31.6 and muscle cramp is also same value because their frequencies are same. Third highest frequent injury is abrasion with a frequency of 7, percentage distribution is 10.4 and injury rate is 36.8%. Blisters, laceration, and rotator cuff are considered as lowest frequent injuries in Basketball as per their ranking and rate of injuries per/100 athletes.

Figure IV-16 Percentage Distribution of Common Injuries in Basketball

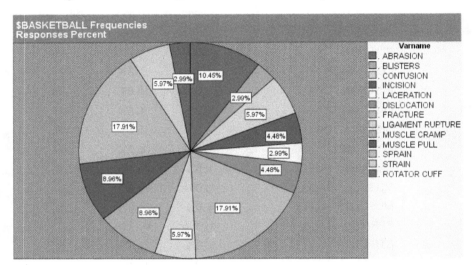

Figure IV-17 Frequencies Distribution of Common Injuries in Basketball

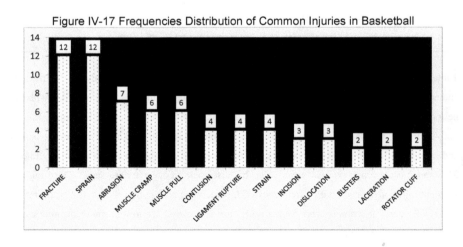

Table IV-20 Frequencies, Percentage and Rate of Common Injuries in Hockey

		Responses		Percent of	Injury Ranking
		N	Percent	Cases	
Injuries	ABRASION	16	19.8%	76.2%	1
	BLISTERS	4	4.9%	19.0%	8
	CONTUSION	15	18.5%	71.4%	2
	INCISION	9	11.1%	42.9%	5
	DISLOCATION	1	1.2%	4.8%	11
	FRACTURE	4	4.9%	19.0%	8
	LIGAMENT RUPTURE	6	7.4%	28.6%	6
	MUSCLE CRAMP	4	4.9%	19.0%	8
	MUSCLE PULL	10	12.3%	47.6%	4
	SPRAIN	10	12.3%	47.6%	4
	TENDINITIS	1	1.2%	4.8%	11
	TENNIS ELBOW	1	1.2%	4.8%	11
Total		**81**	**100.0%**	**385.7%**	

a. Dichotomy group tabulated at value 1.
b. Injury Ranking (1st rank denote highest score) (based on injury rate)
c. Ranks are in descending order

The table 4.20 shows the frequency, percentage distribution and injury rate. Injury rate is also computed. Ranks are in descending order and calculated on the basis of values of injury rate. It is observed that Abrasion is the highest possible injury in Hockey. Frequency of Abrasion is 16 out of total 81, percentage distribution is 19.8% and injury rate is 76.2% respectively. Second most prone injury in Hockey is Contusion. Frequency of Contusion is 15, percentage distribution 18.5% and injury rate is 71.4%. Sprain and Muscle pull is also considerable amount of frequencies and both injuries got 4th rank. Dislocation, Tendinitis and Tennis Elbow found lowest frequent injuries in Hockey. Incision and Ligament Rupture are also frequent injuries noticed with the frequencies 9 (incision), 6 (Ligament Rupture).

Figure IV-18 percentage Distribution of Common Injuries in Hockey

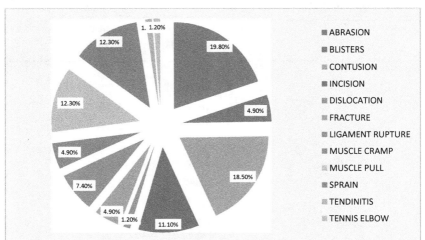

Figure IV-19 Frequencies Distribution of Common Injuries in Hockey

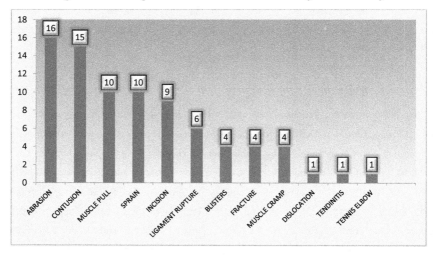

Table IV-21 Frequencies, Percentage and Rate of Common Injuries in Football

		Responses		Percent of Cases	Injury Ranking
		N	Percent		
Injuries	ABRASION	23.00	12.8%	71.9%	1
	SPRAIN	19.00	10.6%	59.4%	2
	CONTUSION	18.00	10.1%	56.2%	3
	MUSCLE CRAMP	17.00	9.5%	53.1%	4
	STRAIN	15.00	8.4%	46.9%	5
	LACERATION	14.00	7.8%	43.8%	6
	BLISTERS	13.00	7.3%	40.6%	7
	LIGAMENT RUPTURE	11.00	6.1%	34.4%	8
	INCISION	9.00	5.0%	28.1%	10
	MUSCLE PULL	9.00	5.0%	28.1%	10
	FRACTURE	8.00	4.5%	25.0%	11
	MENISCUS TEAR	6.00	3.4%	18.8%	12
	DISLOCATION	5.00	2.8%	15.6%	13
	CONCUSSION	4.00	2.2%	12.5%	14
	PUNCTURE WOUND	2.00	1.1%	6.2%	17
	TENDINITIS	2.00	1.1%	6.2%	17
	BACK PAIN	2.00	1.1%	6.2%	17
	ROTATOR CUFF	2.00	1.1%	6.2%	17
Total		**179**	**100.0%**	**559.4%**	

a. Dichotomy group tabulated at value 1.
b. Percentage of Injury cases
c. Injury Ranking (1st rank denote highest score)
d. Ranks are in descending order

Table 4.21 reveals the distribution of common injuries in Football and it was observed that the most common injury in Football is Abrasion with injury rate of 71.9%. Second most frequent injury in Football is Sprain. The injury rate of Sprain is 59.4% and third highest possible injury is Contusion with injury rate of 56.2%. Puncture wound, Tendinitis, Back pain, Rotator Cuff are lowest frequent injuries in Football. A total 179 injuries were recorded during practice and competition of Football players.

Figure IV-20 Percentage Distribution of Common Injuries in Football

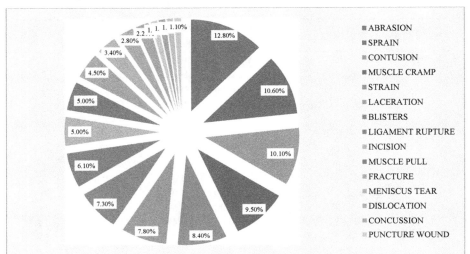

Figure IV-21 Frequencies Distribution of Common Injuries in Football

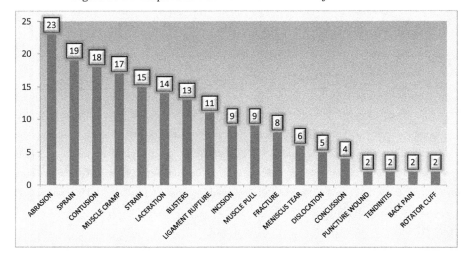

Table IV-22 Frequencies, Percentage and Rate of Common Injuries in Wrestling

		Responses		Percent of	Injury
		N	Percent	Cases	Ranking
Injuries	FRACTURE	10.00	16.7%	38.50	2
	CONTUSION	10.00	16.7%	38.50	2
	SPRAIN	9.00	15.0%	34.60	3
	MUSCLE PULL	8.00	13.3%	30.80	4
	INCISION	6.00	10.0%	23.10	6
	DISLOCATION	6.00	10.0%	23.10	6
	LIGAMENT RUPTURE	5.00	8.3%	19.20	7
	ABRASION	3.00	5.0	11.50	8
	MUSCLE CRAMP	2.00	3.3%	7.70	9
	STRAIN	1.00	1.7%	3.80	10
Total		**60**	**100.0%**	**230.8%**	

a. Dichotomy group tabulated at value 1.
b. Percentage of Injury cases
c. Injury Ranking (1st rank denote highest score) (based on injury rate)
d. Ranks are in descending order

The table 4.22 shows the distribution of frequencies (N), percentage, percentage of cases (IR) and ranking of injuries. As per the obtained data illustrate in table given above most frequent injuries in Wrestling is fracture which percentage is 16.7% and in terms of injury rate (IR) it is 38.50% and got second rank respectively. The Contusion has also same score such as Fracture in wrestling and got same rank. The third most prone injury in Wrestling was Sprain. A total 15% of Sprain measured in wrestlers and IR of Sprain was 34.6% and got third rank. The percentage of muscle pull was 13.3% and IR was 30.8%. Dislocation and Ligament Rupture has also considerable score. Percentage of dislocation was 10% and IR of 23.10% and percentage of Ligament Rupture is 8.3% with IR of 19.20%. Muscle cramp and strain found less inthewind in Wrestling.

Figure IV-22 Percentage Distribution of Common Injuries in wrestling

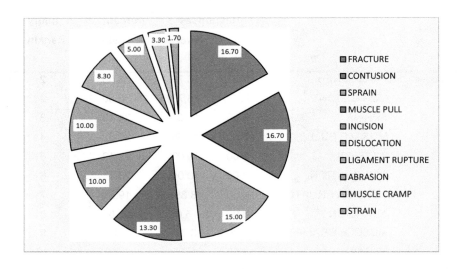

Figure IV-23 Frequency Distribution of Common Injuries in Wrestling

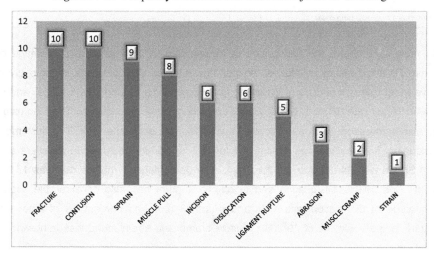

Table IV-23 Frequencies, Percentage and Rate of Common Injuries in weight Lifting

		Responses		Percent	Injury
		N	Percent	of Cases	Ranking
Injury	STRAIN	11	26.8%	55%	1
Ranking	BLISTERS	10	24.4%	50%	2
	MUSCLE PULL	8	19.5%	40%	3
	MUSCLE CRAMP	6	14.6%	30%	4
	CONTUSION	2	4.9%	10%	6
	LIGAMENT RUPTURE	2	4.9%	10%	6
	DISLOCATION	1	2.4%	5%	8
	SPRAIN	1	2.4%	5%	8
Total		**41**	**100.0%**	**205.0%**	

a. Dichotomy group tabulated at value 1.
b. Percentage of Injury cases.
c. Injury Ranking (1st rank denote highest score) (based on injury rate)
d. Ranks are in descending order.

The distribution of frequencies, percentage distribution and rate of injuries in Weight Lifting were reveals in table 4.23 and it was retraced that profuse injury in Weight Lifting was **Strain**. The percentage of strain was 26.8% and percentage of cases (IR) was 55% which was higher score among all injuries and got 1st rank. The second most profuse injury was Blisters found in Weight Lifting. The percentage distribution of Blisters was 24.4% with the Injury Rate of 50% and got 2nd rank respectively. The third most frequent injury was Muscle Pull. The percentage of Muscle pull was 19.5% and injury rate was 40% per 100 athletes with 3rd rank order by. Dislocation and sprain were observed most less deficient injuries in Weight Lifting. The percentage distribution of Dislocation and Sprain was 2.4%, injury Rate was 5% and got Last 8th rank order by.

Figure IV-24 Percentage Distribution of Common Injuries in Weight Lifting

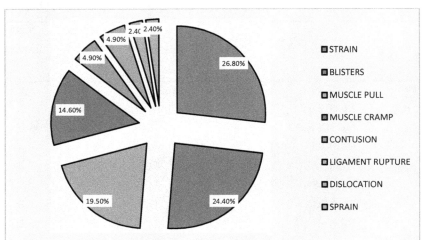

Figure IV-25 Frequency Distribution of Common Injuries in Weight Lifting

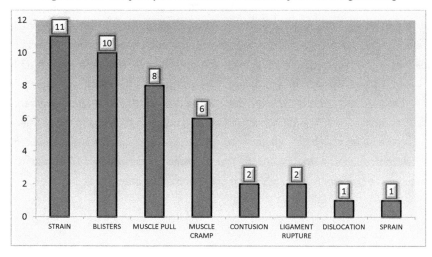

Table IV-24 Frequencies, Percentage and Rate of Common Injuries in Badminton

		Responses		Percent	Injury
		N	Percent	of Cases	Ranking
Injuries	MUSCLE CRAMP	7.00	19.4%	41.20	1
	MUSCLE PULL	6.00	16.7%	35.30	3
	SPRAIN	6.00	16.7%	35.30	3
	ABRASION	5.00	13.9%	29.40	4
	CONTUSION	3.00	8.3%	17.60	6
	TENNIS ELBOW	3.00	8.3%	17.60	6
	FRACTURE	2.00	5.6%	11.80	8
	STRAIN	2.00	5.6%	11.80	8
	LIGAMENT RUPTURE	1.00	2.8%	5.90	10
	TENDINITIS	1.00	2.8%	5.90	10
Total		36	100.0%	211.8%	

a. Dichotomy group tabulated at value 1.
b. Percentage of Injury cases.
c. Injury Ranking (1st rank denote highest score) (based on injury rate)
d. Ranks are in descending order.

The table 4.24 discloses the distribution of percentage, injury rate and ranking and it was retraced that Muscle Cramp was most profuse injury in Badminton. The percentage distribution of Muscle Cramp was 19.4%, IR was 41.20% and got 1st rank and it was lead by Muscle pull. The percentage distribution of muscle pull was 16.7%, injury rate was 35.30% and got 3rd rank. The distribution of Sprain was also same in Badminton with Muscle Pull and got third rank same as Muscle pull. Next frequent injury found in Badminton was Abrasion with percentage distribution of 13.9% and injury rate was 29.4% respectively. Contusion and Tennis Elbow have same occurrence in Badminton. The percentage of Contusion and Tennis Elbow was 8.3% and IR was 17.60% respectively. Ligament Rupture and Tendinitis was found less inthewind injuries in Badminton.

Figure IV-26 Percentage Distribution of Common Injuries in Badminton

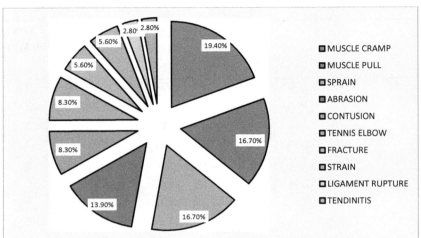

Figure IV-27 Frequency Distribution of Common Injuries in Badminton

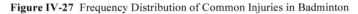
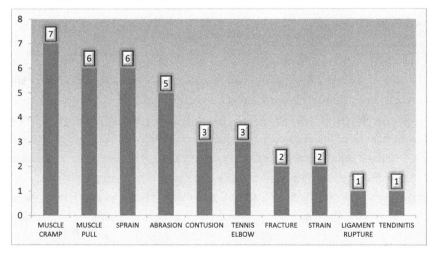

Table IV-25 Frequencies, Percentage and Rate of Common Injuries in Boxing

		Responses		Percent of	Injury Ranking
		N	Percent	Cases	
injuries	CONTUSION	18.00	42.9%	81.80%	1
	MUSCLE PULL	7.00	16.7%	31.80%	2
	FRACTURE	5.00	11.9%	22.70%	3
	LACERATION	4.00	9.5%	18.20%	5
	SPRAIN	4.00	9.5%	18.20%	5
	DISLOCATION	2.00	4.8%	9.10%	6
	ABRSION	1.00	2.4%	4.50%	8
	INCISION	1.00	2.4%	4.50%	8
Total		**42**	**100.0%**	**190.9%**	

a. Dichotomy group tabulated at value 1.
b. Percentage of Injury cases.
c. Injury Ranking (1st rank denote highest score) (based on injury rate)
d. Ranks are in descending order.

The table 4.25 discloses the frequencies, percentage and rage of Common Injuries in Boxing. A total 42 injuries were measured in Boxing. The percentage distribution of **Contusion** is 42.9%, Injury rate was 81.80% and got 1st rank. Percentage distribution of **Muscle** Pull was 16.7% and IR was 31.8% and got 2nd rank. The percentage of **Fracture** was 11.9%, IR 22.07% and Got 3rd rank. The percentage of Laceration and Sprain was 9.5% and Injury Rate was 18.2% respectively. The abrasion and incision were found less inthewind injuries in Boxing. The percentage distribution and Injury rate of Abrasion and Incision were 2.4%±4.50% respectively.

Figure IV-28 Percentage Distribution of Common Injuries in Boxing

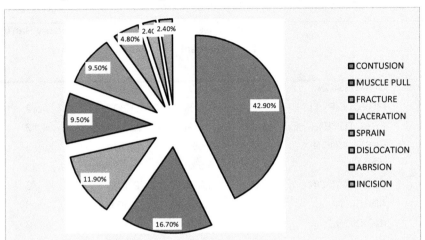

Figure IV-29 Frequency Distribution of Common Injuries in Boxing

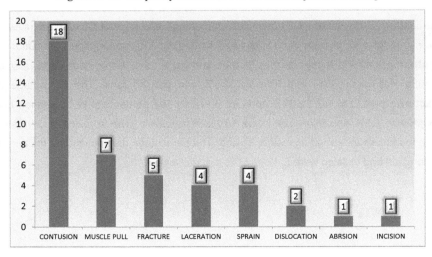

Table IV-26 Frequencies, Percentage and Rate of Common Injuries in Gymnastic

		Responses		Percent of Cases	Injury Ranking
		N	Percent		
Injuries	FRACTURE	12	21.4%	52	1
	ABRASION	10	17.9%	44	2
	BLISTERS	8	14.3%	35	3
	MUSCLE PULL	5	8.9%	22	4
	MUSCLE CRAMP	4	7.1%	17	6
	SPRAIN	4	7.1%	17	6
	CONTUSION	3	5.4%	13	8
	INCISION	3	5.4%	13	8
	DISLOCATION	3	5.4%	13	8
	STRAIN	2	3.6%	9	10
	LIGAMENT RUPTURE	1	1.8%	4	12
	ROTATOR CUFF	1	1.8%	4	12
Total		56	100.0%	243.5%	

a. Dichotomy group tabulated at value 1.
b. Percentage of Injury cases
c. Injury Ranking (1st rank denote highest score) (based on injury rate)
d. Ranks are in descending order.

The table 4.26 discloses the frequencies, percentage and rate of Common Injuries in Gymnastic. A total 56 injuries were measured in Boxing. The percentage distribution of **Fracture** is 21.4%, Injury rate was 52% and got 1st rank. Percentage distribution of **Abrasion** was 17.9% and IR was 44% and got 2nd rank. The percentage of **Blisters** was 14.3%, IR 35% and Got 3rd rank. The percentage of **Muscle Pull** was 8.9% and Injury Rate was 22% respectively. The Ligament Rupture and Rotator Cuff were found less inthewind injuries in Boxing. The percentage distribution and Injury rate of Ligament Rupture and Rotator Cuff were 1.8±4 respectively.

Figure IV-30 Percentage Distribution of Common Injuries in Gymnastic

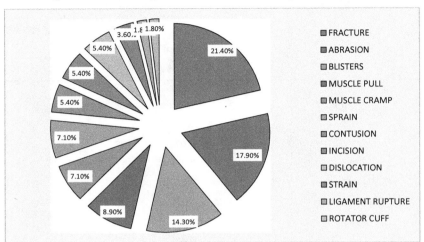

Figure IV-31 Frequency Distribution of Common Injuries in Gymnastic

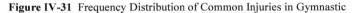

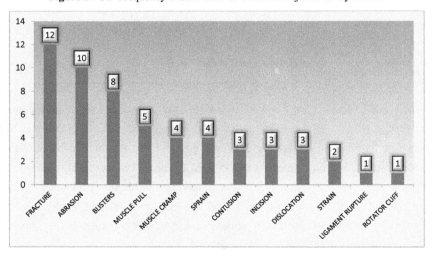

Table IV-27 Frequencies, Percentage and Rate of Common Injuries in Judokas

		Responses		Percent of	Injury
		N	Percent	Cases	Ranking
_a	Abrasion	13	15.5%	86.70	1
	Dislocation	9	10.7%	60.00	2
	Muscle Pull	8	9.5%	53.30	4
	Sprain	8	9.5%	53.30	4
	Contusion	7	8.3%	46.70	6
	Ligament Break	7	8.3%	46.70	6
	Muscle Cramp	7	8.3%	46.70	6
	Fracture	6	7.1%	40.00	8
	Strain	5	6.0%	33.30	9
	Incision	4	4.8%	26.70	11
	Back Pain	4	4.8%	26.70	11
	Blisters	2	2.4%	13.30	13
	MINUSCUS	2	2.4%	13.30	13
	Laceration	1	1.2%	6.70	15
	Rotator Cuff	1	1.2%	6.70	15
Total		84	100.0%	560.0%	

a. Dichotomy group tabulated at value 1.
b. Injury Ranking (1st rank denote highest score) (based on injury rate)
c. Ranks are in descending order.

The table 4.27 discloses the frequencies, percentage and rate of Common Injuries in Judo. It was retraced that 1st rank goes to the **Abrasion** and its percentage distribution is 15.5% and percentage of cases (IR) was 86.70. Second rank goes to Dislocation and its percentage distribution is 10.7% and IR was 60%. Next 4th rank goes to Muscle Pull and its percentage and IR was 9.5±53.30. Laceration and Rotator Cuff found fewer occurrences in Judo and their percentage distribution was 1.2% and Injury Rate was 6.70% respectively.

Figure IV-32 Percentage Distribution of Common Injuries in Judokas

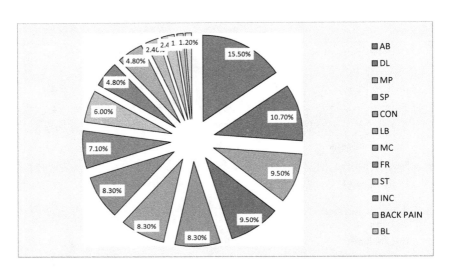

Figure IV-33 Frequency Distribution of Common Injuries in Judokas

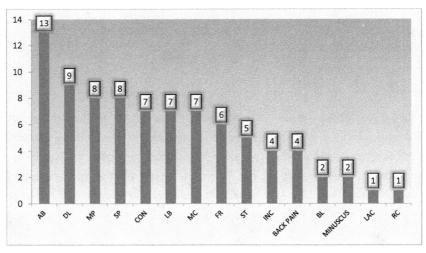

IV.3 Body Parts Associated

Table IV-28 Body Parts Associated with Injuries in Team Games

		Responses		Percent of Cases
		N	Percent	
Body Parts	KNEE	56	13.5%	48.3%
	ANKLE	52	12.5%	44.8%
	ELBOW	39	9.4%	33.6%
	SHOULDER	29	7.0%	25.0%
	THIGH	24	5.8%	20.7%
	CLAF	24	5.8%	20.7%
	EYE BRO	19	4.6%	16.4%
	HAMSTRING MUSCLE	17	4.1%	14.7%
	HAND	16	3.9%	13.8%
	FINGERS	16	3.9%	13.8%
	FOOT	14	3.4%	12.1%
	SHIN	13	3.1%	11.2%
	LUMBER VERTIBRE	12	2.9%	10.3%
	CHIN	11	2.7%	9.5%
	HEAD	9	2.2%	7.8%
	WRIST	7	1.7%	6.0%
	GROWIN MUSCLE	7	1.7%	6.0%
	THUMB	6	1.4%	5.2%
	LOWER LEG	5	1.2%	4.3%
	HEEL	5	1.2%	4.3%
	PALM	4	1.0%	3.4%
	EYE	3	0.7%	2.6%
	FACE	3	0.7%	2.6%
	HIP	3	0.7%	2.6%
	THORASIC VERTIBRE	3	0.7%	2.6%
	FORE HEAD	2	0.5%	1.7%
	NOSE	2	0.5%	1.7%
	COLLER BONE	2	0.5%	1.7%
	PELVIC	2	0.5%	1.7%
	CLEVICLE VERTEBRE	2	0.5%	1.7%
	EAR	1	0.2%	0.9%
	JAW	1	0.2%	0.9%
	CHEST	1	0.2%	0.9%
	UPPER ARM	1	0.2%	0.9%
	LUMBER VERTIBRE	1	0.2%	0.9%
	LCL	1	0.2%	0.9%
	MCL	1	0.2%	0.9%
	ACL	1	0.2%	0.9%
Total		**415**	**100.0%**	**357.8%**

a. Dichotomy group tabulated at value 1.

The associated body parts with sports injuries were disclosed in table 4.28 and it was retraced that the highest probable body part associated with injuries in team games was knee. A total 415 frequencies of body part were measured. Out of that the percentage of **Knee** was 13.5% and IR was 48.3%. Percentage and IR of **Ankle** was 12.5±44.8, **Elbow** was 9.4±33.6, **Shoulder** was 7±25, **Thigh** and **Calf** was 5.8±20.7, **Eyebrow** was 4.6±16.4, **Hamstring** Muscle was 4.1±14.7, **Hand** was 3.9±13.8. Percentage and Injury Rate (IR) of **Fingers** was also 3.9±13.8, percentage and IR of **Foot** was 3.4±12.1. The association of **Shin** with injuries in term of percentage and injury rate (IR) was 3.1± 11.2, **Lumber Vertebrae** was 2.9±10.3, **Chin** was 2.7±9.5 respectively. The percentage distribution and injury rate of **Head** in Team Games was 2.2±7.8. The percentage distribution and injury rate of **Wrist** and **Hamstring** Muscle was same and it was 1.7±6 and **Thumb** was 1.4±5.2. The percentage and injury rate of **Lower Leg** and **Heel** was 1.2±4.3 and percentage distribution and probability of injury occurrence in **Palm** was 1.0±3.4 in Team Games. Percentage distribution and injury rate of **Eye, Face, Hip,** and **Thoracic Vertebrae** in Team Games was 0.7±2.6. Percentage and IR of **Fore Head, Nose, Coller Bone Pelvic Region** and **Clavicle Vertebrae** was 0.5±1.7 respectively. As per illustrate in table 4.28 the lowest inthewind body part were **Ear, Jaw, Chest, Upper Arm, Lumber vertebrae, LCL, MCL, ACL** and their percentage distribution and injury rate were 0.2±0.9 respectively.

Figure IV-34 Percentage Distribution of Injured Body Parts in Team Games

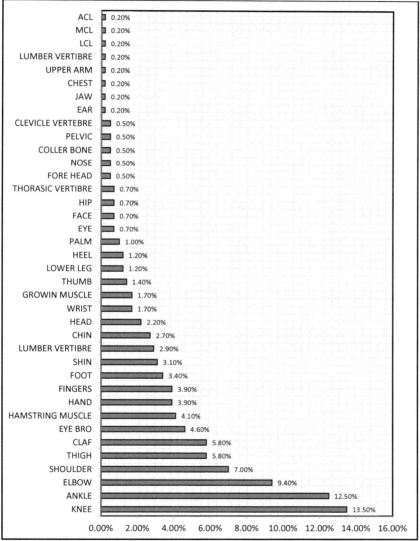

Table IV-29 Body Parts Associated with Injuries in Individual Games

		Responses		Percent of Cases
		N	Percent	
Body Parts	KNEE	56.00	12.8%	40.6%
	SHOULDER	38.00	8.7%	27.5%
	ANKLE	35.00	8.0%	25.4%
	LUMBER VERTEBRAE	32.00	7.3%	23.2%
	ELBOW	24.00	5.5%	17.4%
	FINGERS	18.00	4.1%	13.0%
	THIGH	18.00	4.1%	13.0%
	PALM	17.00	3.9%	12.3%
	FACE	16.00	3.7%	11.6%
	HAMSTRING MUSCLE	14.00	3.2%	10.1%
	WRIST	11.00	2.5%	8.0%
	THUMB	11.00	2.5%	8.0%
	CALF	11.00	2.5%	8.0%
	SHIN	11.00	2.5%	8.0%
	UPPER ARM	10.00	2.3%	7.2%
	NOSE	9.00	2.1%	6.5%
	KNUCKLES	9.00	2.1%	6.5%
	ABDOMEN	8.00	1.8%	5.8%
	HAND	8.00	1.8%	5.8%
	FOREHEAD	7.00	1.6%	5.1%
	EYE	7.00	1.6%	5.1%
	EAR	6.00	1.4%	4.3%
	CHEST	6.00	1.4%	4.3%
	FORE ARM	6.00	1.4%	4.3%
	THORASIC VERTEBRAE	6.00	1.4%	4.3%
	LOWER LEG	5.00	1.1%	3.6%
	FOOT	5.00	1.1%	3.6%
	GROWIN MUSCLE	4.00	0.9%	2.9%
	ACL	4.00	0.9%	2.9%
	EYEBRO	3.00	0.7%	2.2%
	RIBS	3.00	0.7%	2.2%
	LCL	3.00	0.7%	2.2%
	MCL	3.00	0.7%	2.2%
	HEAD	2.00	0.5%	1.4%
	NECK	2.00	0.5%	1.4%
	JAW	2.00	0.5%	1.4%
	LIPS	2.00	0.5%	1.4%
	TOUNGE	1.00	0.2%	0.7%
	COLLER BONE	1.00	0.2%	0.7%
	PLEVIC	1.00	0.2%	0.7%
	HIP	1.00	0.2%	0.7%
	QUADRICEPS	1.00	0.2%	0.7%
	HEEL	1.00	0.2%	0.7%
Total		438	100.0%	317.4%

a. Dichotomy group tabulated at value 1.

The table 4.29 shows the association of body parts with injuries in individual games in term of frequency distribution, percentage and probability of injury occurrence (IR). After analysis the table it was observed that percentage distribution and rate of injury of Knee was also highest in Individual Games and it was 12.8% and IR was 40.6%. The percentage distribution of Shoulder was 8.7% and Injury Rate was 27.5%, percentage and rate of Ankle was 8% and 25.4% (IR). Percentage distribution of Lumber Vertebrae was 7.3% and IR was 23.2%. Percentage of Elbow was 5.5% and IR was 17.4%. Percentage of Fingers and Thigh was 4.1 and IR was 13%. Percentage of Palm was 3.9% and IR was 12.3%. Percentage of Face was 3.7% and IR was 11.6%. Percentage of Hamstring Muscle 3.2% and IR was 10.1%. Percentage of Wrist, Thumb, Calf and Shin was 2.5% and injury rate (IR) was 8%. Percentage of Upper Arm was 2.3% and IR was 7.2%. Percentage of Nose and Knuckles was 2.1% and IR was 6.5%. Percentage distribution of Abdomen and Hand was 1.8% and IR was 5.8%. Percentage of Fore Head and Eye was 1.6% and injury rate (IR) was 5.1%. Percentage distribution of Ear, Chest, Fore Arm, and **Thoracic Vertebrae** was 1.4% and injury rate was 4.3%. Percentage distribution of Lower Leg and Foot in Individual games was 1.1% and injury rate was 3.6%. Percentage distribution of Groin Muscle and Anterior Cruciate Ligament (ACL) was 0.9% and injury rate was 2.9%. Percentage distribution of Eyebrow, Ribs, LCL, and MCL, was 0.7% and Injury rate was 2.2% respectively. Percentage distribution of Head, Neck, Jaw and Lips was 0.5% and injury rate was 1.4% respectively. The lowest frequent injured body parts were Tounge, Collar Bone, Pelvic, Hip, Quadriceps and Heel were 0.2% and injury rate was 0.7% respectively.

Figure IV-35 Percentage Distribution of Injured Body Parts in Individual Games

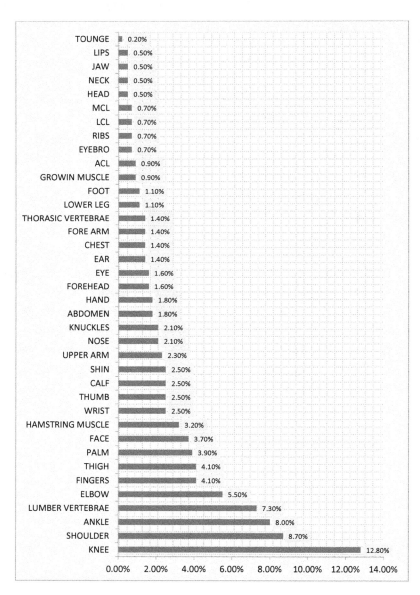

Table IV-30 Body Parts Associated with Injuries in Cricket

		Responses		Percent of Cases
		N	Percent	
BODY-PARTS	ELBOW	8	16.0%	44.4%
	LUMBER VERTEBRAE	7	14.0%	38.9%
	SHOULDER	6	12.0%	33.3%
	FINGERS	5	10.0%	27.8%
	HAMSTRING MUSCLE	5	10.0%	27.8%
	ANKLE	4	8.0%	22.2%
	THIGH	3	6.0%	16.7%
	KNEE	3	6.0%	16.7%
	GROWIN MUSCLE	2	4.0%	11.1%
	SHIN	2	4.0%	11.1%
	FORE HEAD	1	2.0%	5.6%
	FOREARM	1	2.0%	5.6%
	HAND	1	2.0%	5.6%
	PALM	1	2.0%	5.6%
	CALF	1	2.0%	5.6%
Total		50	100.0%	277.8%

a. Dichotomy group tabulated at value 1.

The table no. 4.30 explores the frequency, percentage distribution, and Injury rate (IR) of Cricket. Percentage of Elbow was 16% and IR was 44.4%, Percentage distribution of Lumber Vertebrae was 14% and injury rate was 38.9%. Percentage distribution of Shoulder was 12% and IR was 33.3%. Percentage of Fingers and Hamstring was 10% and injury rate was 27.8%. Percentage of Ankle was 8% and IR was 22.2%. Percentage distribution of Thigh and Knee was 6% and IR was 16.7%. Percentage Distribution of Groin Muscle and Shin was 4% and IR was 11.1%. The lowest inthewind body part were Fore Head, Forearm, Hand, Palm and Calf and their percentage distribution was 2% and injury rate IR was 5.6% respectively.

Figure IV-36 Percentage Distribution of Injured Body Parts in Cricket Players

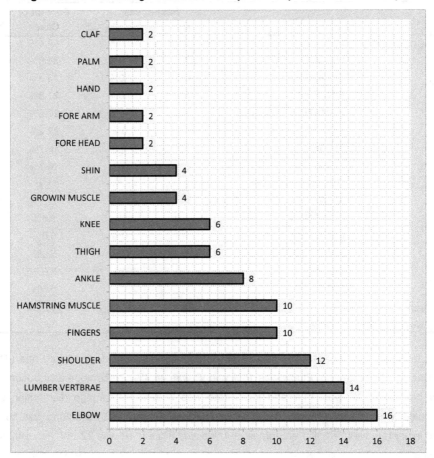

Table IV-31 Body Parts Associated with Injuries in Baseball

		Responses		Percent of Cases
		N	Percent	
BODY PARTS	SHOULDER	12	25.0%	70.6%
	ANKLE	7	14.6%	41.2%
	HAND	4	8.3%	23.5%
	CALF	4	8.3%	23.5%
	EYEBRO	3	6.2%	17.6%
	KNEE	3	6.2%	17.6%
	HEAD	2	4.2%	11.8%
	WRIST	2	4.2%	11.8%
	FINGERS	2	4.2%	11.8%
	THIGH	2	4.2%	11.8%
	EYE	1	2.1%	5.9%
	UPPER ARM	1	2.1%	5.9%
	FORE ARM	1	2.1%	5.9%
	PALM	1	2.1%	5.9%
	SHIN	1	2.1%	5.9%
	CLAVICLE VERTEBRAE	1	2.1%	5.9%
	THORASIC VERTEBRAE	1	2.1%	5.9%
Total		48	100.0%	282.4%

a. Dichotomy group tabulated at value 1.

Association of body parts with injuries in Baseball was disclosed in table 4.31 and it was observed that Percentage distribution of Elbow was 25% and injury rate was 70.6%. Second highest associated body part in Baseball was Ankle and its percentage and IR was 14.6±41.2 respectively. Percentage distribution of Hand and Calf was 4.3% and IR was 23.5% in Baseball. The lowest associated body parts in Baseball was Eye, Upper Arm, Forearm, Palm, Shin, Clavicle Vertebrae and Thoracic Vertebrae and their percentage distribution was 2.1% and injury rate was 5.9% respectively.

Figure IV-37 Percentage Distribution of Injured Body Parts in Baseball Players

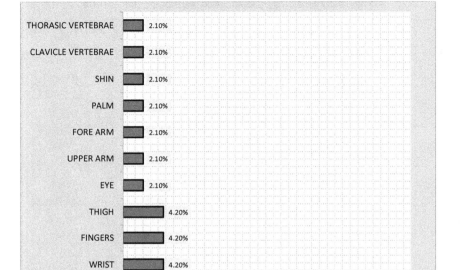

Table IV-32 Body Parts Associated with Injuries Kabaddi

		Responses		Percent of Cases
		N	Percent	
Body Parts[a]	Knee	14	17.7%	63.6%
	Elbow	11	13.9%	50.0%
	Chin	9	11.4%	40.9%
	Ankle	9	11.4%	40.9%
	Eyebrow	6	7.6%	27.3%
	Shoulder	5	6.3%	22.7%
	Thumb	5	6.3%	22.7%
	Fingers	4	5.1%	18.2%
	Wrist	3	3.8%	13.6%
	l-v	3	3.8%	13.6%
	Hand	2	2.5%	9.1%
	Thigh	2	2.5%	9.1%
	Calf	2	2.5%	9.1%
	Nose	1	1.3%	4.5%
	Hip	1	1.3%	4.5%
	c-v	1	1.3%	4.5%
	t-v	1	1.3%	4.5%
Total		**79**	**100.0%**	**359.1%**

a. Dichotomy group tabulated at value 1.

The table 4.32 evident the frequencies, percentage distribution and injury rate of Kabaddi players. Only three highest and three lowest parts were described within the table. Percentage of Knee was 17.7% and IR was 63.6%. Percentage of Elbow was 13.9% and IR was 50%. Percentage of Chin was 11.4% and IR was 40.9%. The lowest inthewind body parts were Nose, HIP Clavicle Vertebrae, and Thoracic Vertebrae and their percentage distribution was 1.3% and Injury Rate (IR) was 4.5% respectively.

Figure IV-38 Percentage Distribution of Injured Body Parts in Kabaddi Players

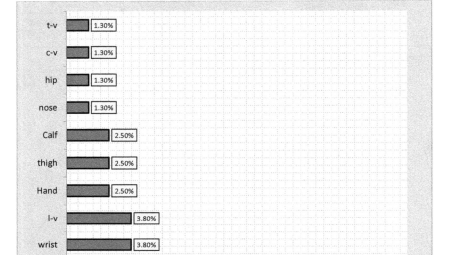

Table IV-33 Body Parts Associated with Injuries in Basketball

| | | Responses | | Percent of |
		N	Percent	Cases
BODY	ANKLE	9	25.0%	64.3%
PARTS[a]	KNEE	7	19.4%	50.0%
	ELBOW	4	11.1%	28.6%
	SHOULDER	2	5.6%	14.3%
	HAND	2	5.6%	14.3%
	THIGH	2	5.6%	14.3%
	EYE	1	2.8%	7.1%
	EYE BRO	1	2.8%	7.1%
	NOSE	1	2.8%	7.1%
	WRIST	1	2.8%	7.1%
	THUMB	1	2.8%	7.1%
	HIP	1	2.8%	7.1%
	GROWIN MUSCLE	1	2.8%	7.1%
	HAMSTRING MUSCLE	1	2.8%	7.1%
	CALF	1	2.8%	7.1%
	LUMBER VERTEBRAE	1	2.8%	7.1%
Total		**36**	**100.0%**	**257.1%**

a. Dichotomy group tabulated at value 1.

The table 4.33 evident the frequencies, percentage distribution and injury rate of Basketball players. Only three highest and three lowest parts were described within the table. Percentage of Ankle was 25% and IR was 64.3%. Percentage of Knee was 19.4% and IR was 50%. Percentage of Elbow was 11.1% and IR was 28.6%.

The lowest inthewind body parts were Hamstring Muscle, Calf and Lumber Vertebrae their percentage distribution was 2.8% and Injury Rate (IR) was 7.1% respectively.

Figure IV-39 Percentage Distribution of Injured Body Parts in Basketball Players

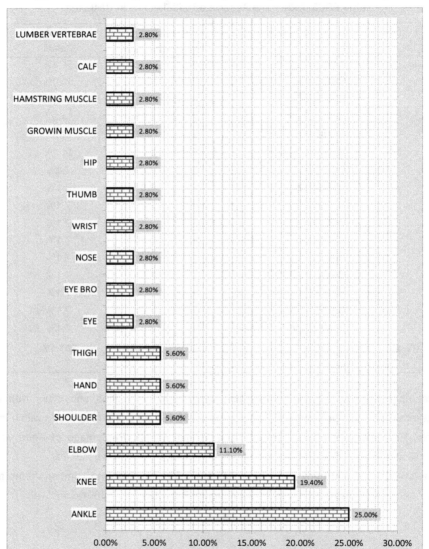

Table IV-34 Body Parts Associated with Injuries in Hockey

		Responses		Percent of Cases
		N	Percent	
BODY	KNEE	9	13.0%	60.0%
PARTS[a]	ELBOW	7	10.1%	46.7%
	HAM. MUS	6	8.7%	40.0%
	ANKLE	6	8.7%	40.0%
	EYE BRO	5	7.2%	33.3%
	SHIN	5	7.2%	33.3%
	CALF	4	5.8%	26.7%
	FOOT	4	5.8%	26.7%
	THIGH	3	4.3%	20.0%
	CHIN	2	2.9%	13.3%
	SHOULDER	2	2.9%	13.3%
	HAND	2	2.9%	13.3%
	FINGERS	2	2.9%	13.3%
	PELVIC	2	2.9%	13.3%
	GROWIN MUSCLE	2	2.9%	13.3%
	HAMSTRING MUSCLE	1	1.4%	6.7%
	COLLER BONE	1	1.4%	6.7%
	UPPER ARM	1	1.4%	6.7%
	PALM	1	1.4%	6.7%
	LOWER LEG	1	1.4%	6.7%
	LCL	1	1.4%	6.7%
	MCL	1	1.4%	6.7%
	ACL	1	1.4%	6.7%
Total		**69**	**100.0%**	**460.0%**

a. Dichotomy group tabulated at value 1.

The table 4.34 evident the frequencies, percentage distribution and injury rate of Hockey players. Only three highest and three lowest parts were described within the table. Percentage of Knee was 13%% and IR was 60%. Percentage of Elbow was 10.1% and IR was 46.7%. Percentage of Hamstring Muscle was 8.7% and IR was 40%.

The lowest inthewind body parts were LCL, MCL and ACL and their percentage distribution was 1.4% and IR was 6.7% respectively.

Figure IV-40 Percentage Distribution of Injured Body Parts in Hockey Players

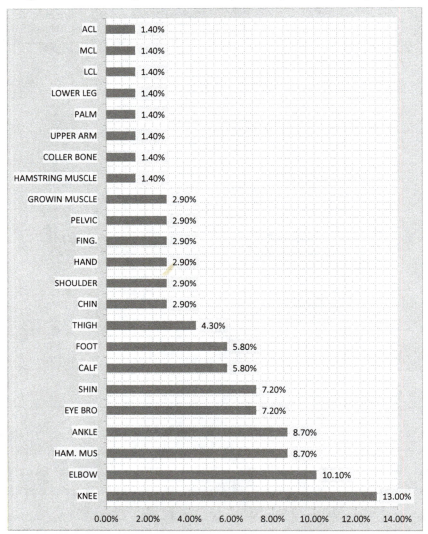

Table IV-35 Body Parts Associated with Injuries in Football

		Responses		Percent of Cases
		N	Percent	
BODY PARTS[a]	KNEE	21	15.1%	67.7%
	ANKLE	17	12.2%	54.8%
	THIGH	12	8.6%	38.7%
	CALF	12	8.6%	38.7%
	FOOT	10	7.2%	32.3%
	ELBOW	9	6.5%	29.0%
	HEAD	5	3.6%	16.1%
	EYE BRO	5	3.6%	16.1%
	SHOULDER	5	3.6%	16.1%
	HAND	5	3.6%	16.1%
	HAMSTRING MUSCLE	5	3.6%	16.1%
	SHIN	5	3.6%	16.1%
	HEEL	5	3.6%	16.1%
	LOWER LEG	4	2.9%	12.9%
	FACE	3	2.2%	9.7%
	FINGERS	3	2.2%	9.7%
	GROWOM MUSCLE	2	1.4%	6.5%
	FORE HEAD	1	0.7%	3.2%
	EYE	1	0.7%	3.2%
	EAR	1	0.7%	3.2%
	JAW	1	0.7%	3.2%
	CHEST	1	0.7%	3.2%
	COLLER BONE	1	0.7%	3.2%
	WRIST	1	0.7%	3.2%
	PALM	1	0.7%	3.2%
	HIP	1	0.7%	3.2%
	THORASIC VERTEBRAE	1	0.7%	3.2%
	LUMBER VERTEBRAE	1	0.7%	3.2%
Total		139	100.0%	448.4%

a. Dichotomy group tabulated at value 1.

The table 4.35 evident the frequencies, percentage distribution and injury rate of Football players. Only three highest and three lowest parts were described within the table. Percentage of Knee was 15.1% and IR was 67.7%. Percentage of Ankle was 8.6% and IR was 54.8%. Percentage of Thigh was 8.6% and IR was 38.7%.

The lowest inthewind body parts Hip, Thoracic and Lumber Vertebrae their percentage distribution was 0.7% and Injury Rate (IR) was 3.2% respectively

Figure IV-41 Percentage Distribution of Injured Body Parts in Football Players

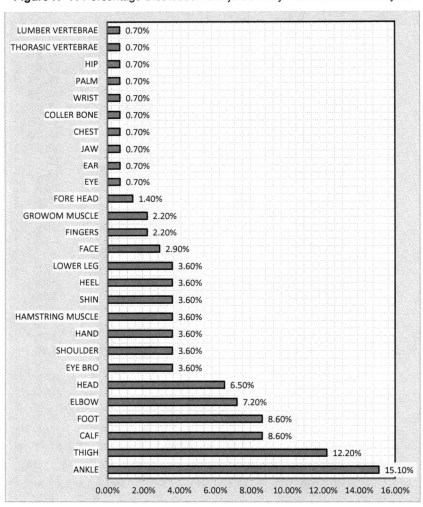

Table IV-36 Body Parts Associated with Injuries in Wrestlers

		Responses		Percent of Cases
		N	Percent	
BODY PARTS	KNEE	13	18.3%	59.1%
	ELBOW	7	9.9%	31.8%
	FINGERS	6	8.5%	27.3%
	ANKLE	6	8.5%	27.3%
	EAR	4	5.6%	18.2%
	SHOULDER	4	5.6%	18.2%
	THUMB	4	5.6%	18.2%
	LUMBER VERTEBRAE	4	5.6%	18.2%
	RIBS	3	4.2%	13.6%
	HEAD	2	2.8%	9.1%
	NECK	2	2.8%	9.1%
	EBRO	2	2.8%	9.1%
	NOSE	2	2.8%	9.1%
	FACE	2	2.8%	9.1%
	FORE HEAD	1	1.4%	4.5%
	EYE	1	1.4%	4.5%
	CHEST	1	1.4%	4.5%
	UPPER ARM	1	1.4%	4.5%
	FORE ARM	1	1.4%	4.5%
	HAND	1	1.4%	4.5%
	PELVIC	1	1.4%	4.5%
	HAMSTRING MUSCLE	1	1.4%	4.5%
	FOOT	1	1.4%	4.5%
	LCL	1	1.4%	4.5%
Total		71	100.0%	322.7%

a. Dichotomy group tabulated at value 1.

The table 4.36 evident the frequencies, percentage distribution and injury rate of Wrestlers. Only three highest and three lowest parts were described within the table. Percentage of Knee was 18.3% and IR was 59.1%. Percentage of Elbow was 9.9% and IR was 31.8%. Percentage of Fingers was 8.5% and IR was 27.3%.

The lowest inthewind body parts were Hamstring, Foot, and LCL and their percentage distribution was 1.4% and Injury Rate (IR) was 4.5% respectively

Figure IV-42 Percentage Distribution of Injured Body Parts in Wrestlers

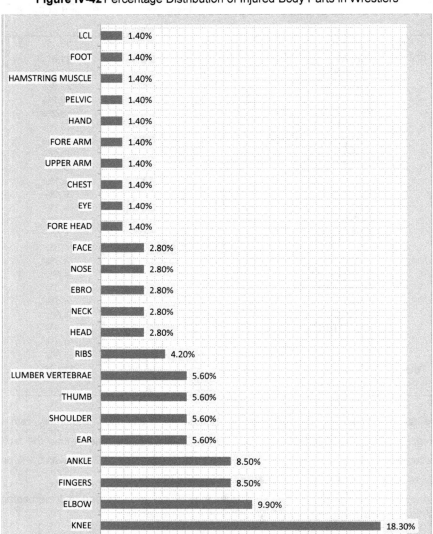

Table IV-37 Body Parts Associated with Injuries in Weight Lifting

		Responses		Percent of Cases
		N	**Percent**	
BODY PARTS[a]	LUMBER-VERTEBRAE	8	22.2%	57.1%
	PALM	6	16.7%	42.9%
	KNEE	6	16.7%	42.9%
	SHOULDER	4	11.1%	28.6%
	THIGH	3	8.3%	21.4%
	ELBOW	2	5.6%	14.3%
	WRIST	2	5.6%	14.3%
	THORASIC-VERTEBRAE	2	5.6%	14.3%
	UPPER ARM	1	2.8%	7.1%
	QUADRICEPS	1	2.8%	7.1%
	HAMSTRING MUSCLE	1	2.8%	7.1%
Total		**36**	**100.0%**	**257.1%**

a. Dichotomy group tabulated at value 1.

The table 4.37 evident the frequencies, percentage distribution and injury rate of Weight Lifters. Only three highest and three lowest parts were described within the table. The **First** Highest associated and Injury Probable body part in Weight Litter was Lumber Vertebrae or Low Back. Percentage of Low Back was 22.2% and IR was 57.1%. **Second** Highest Probable body part was Palm. Percentage of Palm was 16.7% and IR was 42.9%. **Third** highest associated and injury probable body parts was Knee. Percentage of Knee was 16.7% and IR was 42.9%.

The lowest inthewind body parts were Upper arm, Quadriceps and Hamstring Muscle and their percentage distribution was 2.8% and Injury Rate (IR) was 7.1% respectively.

Figure IV-43 Percentage Distribution of Injured Body Parts in Weight Lifters

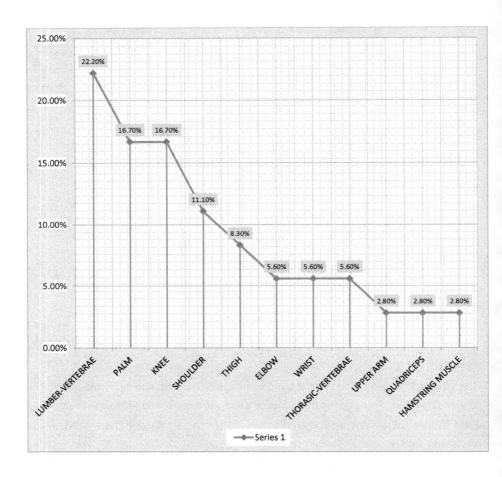

Table IV-38 Body Parts Associated with Injuries in Badminton Players

		Responses		Percent of Cases
		N	Percent	
BODY	KNEE	7	15.6%	36.8%
PARTS[a]	ANKLE	7	15.6%	36.8%
	SHOULDER	6	13.3%	31.6%
	UPPER ARM	5	11.1%	26.3%
	ELBOW	3	6.7%	15.8%
	THIGH	3	6.7%	15.8%
	WRIST	2	4.4%	10.5%
	HAMSTRING MUSCLE	2	4.4%	10.5%
	LOWER LEG	2	4.4%	10.5%
	SHIN	2	4.4%	10.5%
	HAND	1	2.2%	5.3%
	FINGERS	1	2.2%	5.3%
	GROWIN MUSCLE	1	2.2%	5.3%
	CALF	1	2.2%	5.3%
	L-V*	1	2.2%	5.3%
	ACL	1	2.2%	5.3%
Total		45	100.0%	236.8%

a. Dichotomy group tabulated at value 1.

b. L-V Denotes Lumber Vertebrae

The table 4.38 evident the frequencies, percentage distribution and injury rate of Badminton Players. Only three highest and three lowest parts were described within the table.   The **First** Highest associated and Injury Probable body part in Shutters was Knee. Percentage of Knee was 15.6% and IR was 36.8%. **Second** Highest Probable body part was Ankle. Percentage of Ankle was 15.6% and IR was 36.8%. **Third** highest associated and injury probable body parts was Shoulder. Percentage of Shoulder was 13.3% and IR was 31.6%.

The lowest inthewind body parts were Calf, L-V and ACL and their percentage distribution was 2.2% and Injury Rate (IR) was 5.3% respectively.

Figure IV-44 Percentage Distribution of Injured Body Parts in Badminton Players

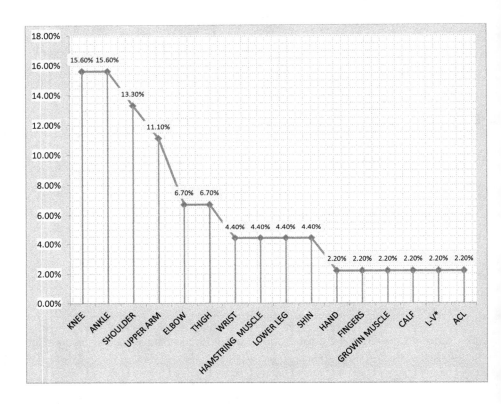

Table IV-39 Body Parts Associated with Injuries in Boxers

		Responses		Percent of
		N	Percent	Cases
BODY	KNUCKLES	9	15.3%	42.9%
PARTS[a]	NOSE	7	11.9%	33.3%
	THUMB	7	11.9%	33.3%
	SHOULDER	6	10.2%	28.6%
	L-V*	6	10.2%	28.6%
	EYE	5	8.5%	23.8%
	ELBOW	5	8.5%	23.8%
	ANKLE	3	5.1%	14.3%
	EAR	2	3.4%	9.5%
	JAW	2	3.4%	9.5%
	FINGERS	2	3.4%	9.5%
	EYE BRO	1	1.7%	4.8%
	FACE	1	1.7%	4.8%
	TOUNGE	1	1.7%	4.8%
	WRIST	1	1.7%	4.8%
	PALM	1	1.7%	4.8%
	Total	**59**	**100.0%**	**281.0%**

a. Dichotomy group tabulated at value 1.
B*. L-V Denotes Lumber Vertebrae

The table 4.39 evident the frequencies, percentage distribution and injury rate of Boxers. Only three highest and three lowest parts were described within the table. The **First** Highest associated and Injury Probable body part in Boxers was Knuckles. Percentage of Knuckles was 15.3% and IR was 42.9%. **Second** Highest Probable body part was Nose. Percentage of Nose was 11.3% and IR was 33.3%. **Third** highest associated and injury probable body parts was Thumb. Percentage of Thumb was 11.9% and IR was 33.3%.

The lowest inthewind body parts were Tounge, Wrist and Palm their percentage distribution was 1.7and Injury Rate (IR) was 4.8% respectively.

Figure IV-45 Percentage Distribution of Injured Body Parts in Boxers

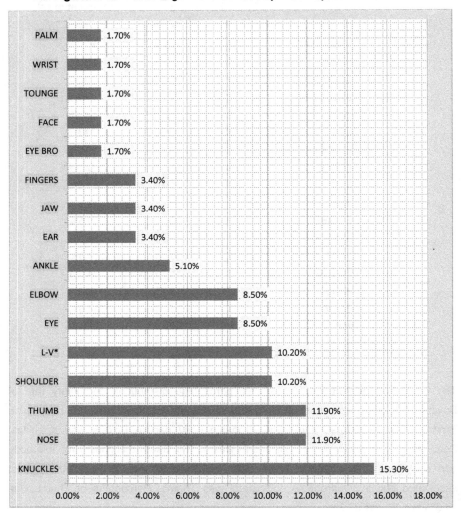

Table IV-40 Body Parts Associated with Injuries in Gymnasts

| | | Responses | | Percent of |
		N	Percent	Cases
BODY	SHOULDER	6	12.8%	33.3%
PARTS[a]	HAND	6	12.8%	33.3%
	PALM	5	10.6%	27.8%
	KNEE	5	10.6%	27.8%
	ANKLE	4	8.5%	22.2%
	LOWER LEG	3	6.4%	16.7%
	UPPER ARM	2	4.3%	11.1%
	ELBOW	2	4.3%	11.1%
	WRIST	2	4.3%	11.1%
	FINGERS	2	4.3%	11.1%
	THIGH	2	4.3%	11.1%
	L-V*	2	4.3%	11.1%
	EYE	1	2.1%	5.6%
	COLLER BONE	1	2.1%	5.6%
	HIP	1	2.1%	5.6%
	HEEL	1	2.1%	5.6%
	T-V*	1	2.1%	5.6%
	MCL*	1	2.1%	5.6%
Total		**47**	**100.0%**	**261.1%**

a. Dichotomy group tabulated at value 1.
* L-V (Lumber Vertebrae)
*T-V (Thoracic Vertebrae)
*MCL(Medial Collateral Ligament

The table 4.40 evident the frequencies, percentage distribution and injury rate of Gymnasts. Only three highest and three lowest parts were described within the table. The **First** Highest associated and Injury Probable body part in Gymnasts was Shoulders. Percentage of Shoulders was 12.8% and IR was 33.3%. **Second** Highest Probable body part was Hand. Percentage of Hand was 12.8% and IR was 33.3%.

Third highest associated and injury probable body parts was Palm. Percentage of Palm was 10.6% and IR was 27.8%.

The lowest inthewind body parts were Heel, T-V, and MCL and their percentage distribution was 2.1and Injury Rate (IR) was 5.6% respectively.

Figure IV-46 Percentage Distribution of Injured Body Parts in Gymnasts

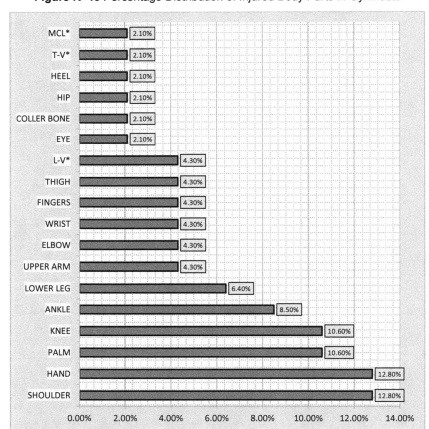

Table IV-41 Body Parts Associated with Injuries in Judo

		Responses		Percent of Cases
		N	Percent	
BODY PARTS[a]	KNEE	15	11.7%	78.9%
	FACE	13	10.2%	68.4%
	ANKLE	11	8.6%	57.9%
	SHOULDER	9	7.0%	47.4%
	ABDOMEN	8	6.2%	42.1%
	THIGH	7	5.5%	36.8%
	CALF	7	5.5%	36.8%
	FORE HEAD	6	4.7%	31.6%
	FINGERS	6	4.7%	31.6%
	L-V*	6	4.7%	31.6%
	CHEST	5	3.9%	26.3%
	SHIN	5	3.9%	26.3%
	ELBOW	4	3.1%	21.1%
	FORE ARM	4	3.1%	21.1%
	WRIST	4	3.1%	21.1%
	HAMSTRING MUSCLE	4	3.1%	21.1%
	LIPS	2	1.6%	10.5%
	PALM	2	1.6%	10.5%
	GROWIN MUSCLE	2	1.6%	10.5%
	FOOT	2	1.6%	10.5%
	T-V*	2	1.6%	10.5%
	LCL*	2	1.6%	10.5%
	MCL*	2	1.6%	10.5%
Total		**128**	**100.0%**	**673.7%**

a. Dichotomy group tabulated at value 1.
* L-V (Lumber Vertebrae)
* T-V (Thoracic Vertebrae)
* LCL (Lateral Collateral Ligament)
* MCL (Medial Collateral Ligament

The table 4.41 evident the frequencies, percentage distribution and injury rate of Judokas. Only three highest and three lowest parts were described within the table. The **First** Highest associated and Injury Probable body part in Judokas was Knee. Percentage of Knee was 11.7% and IR was 78.9%. **Second** Highest Probable body part was Face. Percentage of Face was 10.2% and IR was 68.4%. **Third** highest associated and injury probable body parts was Ankle. Percentage of Ankle was 8.6% and IR was 57.9%.

The lowest inthewind body parts were T-V, LCL and MCL their percentage distribution was 1.6% and Injury Rate (IR) was 10.5% respectively.

Figure IV-47 Percentage Distribution of Injured Body Parts in Judo

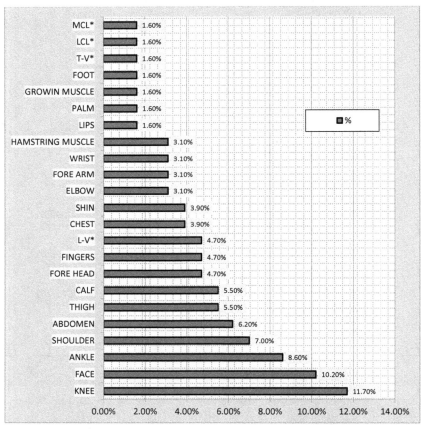

IV.4 Classification of Injury Severity

Table IV-42 Classification of Injury severity in Team and Individual Sports

	Team Game				Individual Game		
	Mean	**Minimum**	**Maximum**		**Mean**	**Minimum**	**Maximum**
Meniscus tear	150.00	120	180	Meniscus tear	227.50	90	365
Ligament Rupture	129.26	15	365	Ligament Rupture	129.38	60	400
Fracture	63.61	4	180	Dislocation	83.00	7	365
concussion	63.33	10	120	Fracture	78.43	2	365
Low back pain	60.00	60	60	Low back pain	75.55	4	365
Jerk	45.60	5	180	Shin pain	31.50	15	60
Tendinitis	34.60	2	150	Rotator cuff	30.00	30	30
Dislocation	34.53	6	90	Muscle pull	18.56	2	180
Puncture wound	32.50	10	60	Jerk	16.64	5	60
Tooth break	28.00	10	60	Sprain	14.60	2	60
Rotator cuff	23.75	2	120	Contusion	14.13	2	90
Sprain	18.41	1	90	Strain	12.73	2	60
Muscle pull	14.08	2	90	Tennis elbow	11.67	10	15
Incision	13.45	1	120	Incision	10.00	2	45
Laceration	11.75	1	60	Muscle cramp	8.80	1	21
Muscle cramp	9.31	1	30	Blisters	7.63	2	30
Strain	8.45	1	30	Laceration	7.57	2	15
Contusion	6.09	1	20	Tendinitis	6.00	5	7
Blisters	4.18	1	7	Abrasion	5.15	2	30
Abrasion	4.16	1	30	Tooth break	.00	0	0
Muscle Tear	-	-	-	Muscle Tear	-	-	-
Tennis elbow	-	-	-	Puncture wound	-	-	-
Shin pain	.00	0	0	concussion	-	-	-

*Injury Severity Based on total days lost from competition and practice due to injury.
*Data arranged in descending order.

The table 4.42 demonstrates the mean score of injury severity in team and individual sports. The score of injury severity was based total days lost from competition and practice due to injury occurred. In the table given above the data were arranged in descending order. After analysis the table it was observed that the most severe injury in **Team Games** was **Ligament rupture** and **Meniscus tear** their respective mean score was 129.26±150 days. Next severe injuries in team games were Fracture and Concussion and their mean score were **Fracture** and **Concussion** and their mean score were 63.61±63.33 days. The mean score of **Low Back Pain** and **Jerk** were 60±45.60 days. The Mean score of **Tendinitis** and **Dislocation** were 34.60±34.53 days respectively. The severity score of **Puncture Wound** and **Tooth Break** were 32.50±28 days. The mean score of severity of **Rotator Cuff** and **Sprain** were 23.75±18.41days. **Muscle Pull** and **Incision** were 14.08±13.45 days. **Laceration** and **Muscle Cramp** were 11.75±9.31 days. The Strain and Contusion were 8.45±6.09 days and the mean score of **Blisters** and **Abrasion** were 4.18±4.16 days. No **Muscle Tear** and **Tennis Elbow** were observed in Team Games during data collection. So, the outputs of severity were not computed by SPSS. No rest was taken on **Shin Pain** by Team Game players.

In **Individual Games** highest severe injury were also **Meniscus Tear** and **Ligament Rupture** with the mean score of 227.50±129.26 days. Mean score of **Dislocation** and **Fracture** were 83±78.43 days. Mean score of **Low Back Pain** and **Shin Pain** were 75.55±31.50 days. **Rotator Cuff** and **Muscle Pull** were 30±18.56 days. **Jerk** and **Sprain** were 16.64±14.60 days. **Contusion** and **Strain** were 14.13±12.73 days. **Tennis Elbow** and **Incision** were 11.67±10 days. **Muscle Cramps** and **Blisters** were 8.80±7.63 days. **Laceration** and **Tendinitis** were 7.57±6 days and the mean score of severity of **Abrasion** was 5.15 days respectively. No sufficient data of **Muscle Tear, Puncture Wound** and **Concussion** were found to compute the mean score of injury severity of these injuries.

Figure IV-48 Mean Score of Injury Severity of Team and Individual Sports Competitions

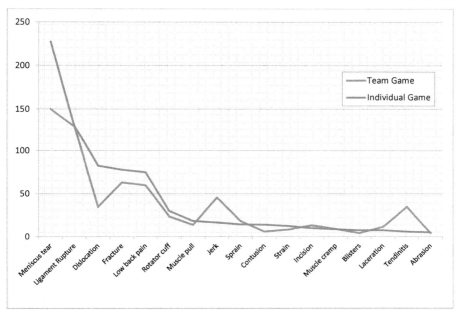

Table IV-43 Classification of Injury severity in Each Game

	Cricket	Baseball	Kabaddi	Basketball	Hockey	Football	Wrestling	Weight lifting	Badminton	Boxing	Gymnastic	Judo
Abrasion	2.83	4.40	2.50	4.29	3	6	4.50	-	3.40	-	7.80	-
Blisters	2	3.33	-	4.50	4.75	4.33	-	6.17	-	-	9	2
Contusion	6	3.50	8.40	4.67	3.83	6.93	9.38	45	3.33	10.67	7	17.25
Incision	-	-	20	32.5	10	3.63	5.67	-	-	10	20.33	5
Laceration	-	3	8.50	7	-	13.64	7	-	-	10.67	-	-
Dislocation	-	30	40.33	17	30	36.40	69	30	-	57.50	62.67	82.83
Fracture	30	61.33	91.11	70	23.33	49.71	70	-	120	26.40	117.2	34
Tooth break	-	-	-	35	-	14	-	-	-	-	-	-
Jerk	49.50	-	30	-	-	-	10.50	52.50	7.20	-	-	-
Ligament rupture	120	63.75	100	171	172.5	127	75	60	90-	-	365	227.50
Muscle tear	-	-	-	-	-	-	-	-	-	-	-	-
Muscle camp	4.50	17.50	20	5.67	22	3.92	15	9	5	-	11.50	1.50
Muscle pull	12.43	16.70	15.67	9.40	4	21.86	18.80	10.40	8	7.33	5.33	10.80
Puncture wound	60	15	-	-	-	27.50	-	-	-	-	-	-
Sprain	9.20	18.36	19.25	16.59	29.67	18.39	24.88	7	7.67	16	9	15.40
Strain	8.67	10	20	15	-	7.07	5	21.25	5.50	-	30	3
Tendinitis	7	-	-	7	150	4.50	-	-	5	-	-	7
Tennis elbow	-	-	-	-	-	-	-	-	11.67	-	-	-
Rotator cuff	-	29	-	14	-	2	-	-	-	-	30	30
Low back pain	-	-	-	-	-	60	-	31.67	-	53.50	-	212.5
Meniscus tear	-	-	-	-	-	150	90	-	-	-	-	365
Shin pain	-	-	-	-	-	-	-	-	-	-	-	-
concussion	-	-	-	-	-	63.33	-	-	-	-	-	-

Injury Severity Based on total days lost from competition and practice due to injury.

Figure IV-49 Mean Score of Injury Severity in Cricket

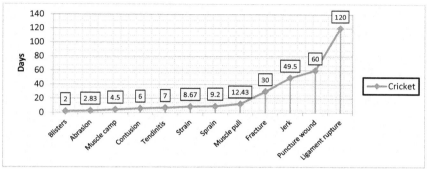

Figure IV-50 Mean Score of Injury Severity in Baseball

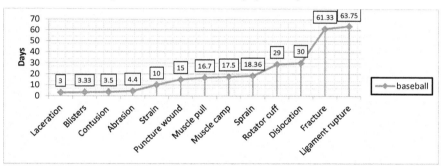

Figure IV-51 Mean Score of Injury Severity in Kabaddi

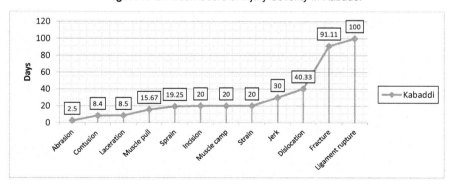

Figure IV-52 Mean Score of Injury Severity in Basketball

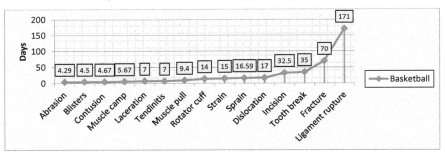

Figure IV-53 Mean Score of Injury Severity in Hockey

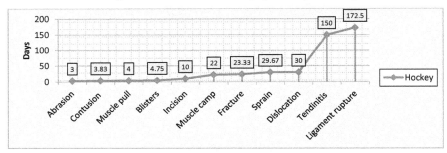

Figure IV-54 Mean Score of Injury Severity in Football

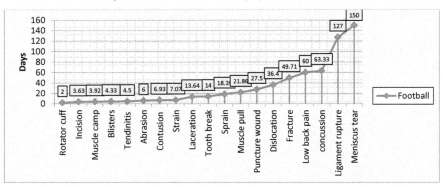

Figure IV-55 Mean Score of Injury Severity in Wrestling

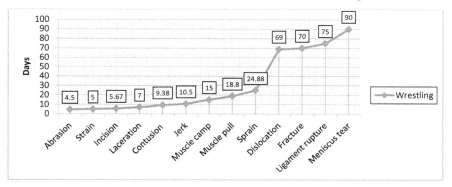

Figure IV-56 Mean Score of Injury Severity in Weight Lifting

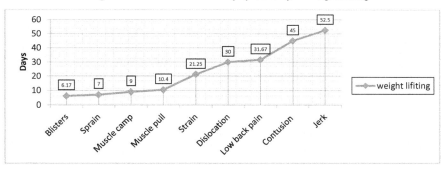

Figure IV-57 Mean Score of Injury Severity in Badminton

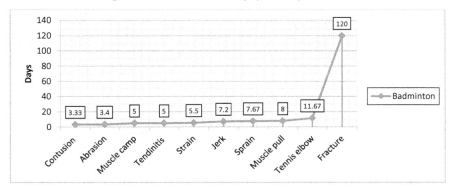

Figure IV-58 Mean Score of Injury Severity in Boxing

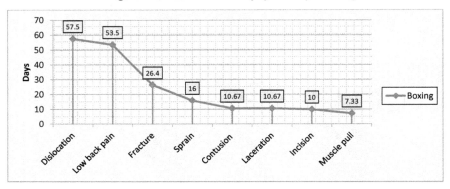

Figure IV-59 Mean Score of Injury Severity in Gymnastic

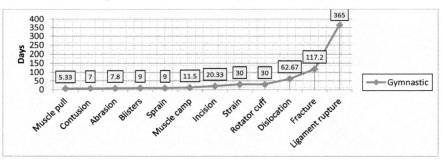

Figure IV-60 Mean Score of Injury Severity in Judo

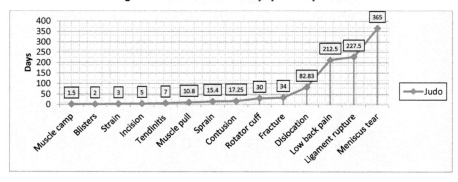

IV.5 Injuries in Match or Training

Table IV-44 Percentage Distribution of Match and Training Injuries in Team and individual Games

		N	Percentage
Team Games	Match Injuries	260	56.76
	Training Injuries	198	43.24
	Total	**458**	**100**
Individual Games	Match Injuries	87	33.20
	Training Injuries	175	66.79
	Total	**262**	**100**

The table 4.44 reveals the frequencies and percentage distribution of match and training injuries in Team and Individual games and it was retraced that a total 458 injures were noticed in Team Games. Out of that 56.76% injuries occurred during match or competition and 43.24 injuries occurred during training. In Individual Games a total 262 injuries were measured. Out of the following 33.20% were occurred in match and 66.79% injuries occurred during training or practice.

Table IV-45 Game wise Percentage Distribution of Match and Training Injuries

Team Games	Match Injuries		Training Injuries		Individual Games	Match Injuries		Training Injuries	
	N	%	N	%		N	%	N	%
Cricket	12	4.61%	14	7.07%	Wrestling	17	19.54	13	7.42%
Baseball	32	12.30%	36	18.18%	Weight Lifting	2	2.29	18	10.28%
Kabaddi	12	4.61%	14	7.07%	Badminton	9	10.34	11	6.28%
Basketball	32	12.30%	34	17.17%	Boxing	5	5.74	22	12.57%
Hockey	63	24.33%	27	13.63%	Gymnastic	10	11.49	49	28%
Football	109	41.92%	73	36.86%	Judo	44	50.57	62	35.42%
Total	**260**	**100%**	**198**	**100%**	**Total**	**87**	**100**	**175**	**100**

The table 4.45 illustrates the frequencies and percentage distribution of each selected game and after analysis the table it was observed that percentage of match and training injuries in Cricket were 4.61±7.07, in Baseball percentage distribution of match and training injuries were 12.30±18.18, in Kabaddi 4.61±7.07, in Basketball 12.30±17.17, in Hockey 24.33±13.63, and in Football percentage distribution of match and training injuries were 41.92±36.86 respectively. In Individual Games the percentage distribution of match and training injuries of Wrestling were 19.54±7.42, in Weight Lifting 2.29±10.28, in Badminton 10.34±6.28 percent, in Boxing 5.74±12.57, in Gymnastic 11.49±28 percent, in Judo percentage distribution of match and training injuries were 50.57±35.42 respectively.

Figure IV-61 Match and Training Injuries in Team and Individual Games

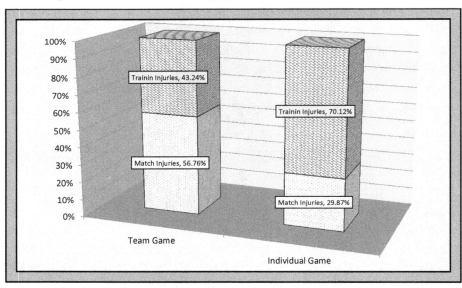

Figure IV-62 Match and Training Injuries in Team Games

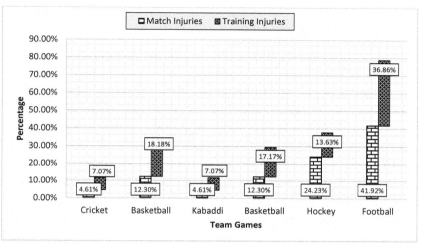

Figure IV-63 Match and Training Injuries in Individual Games

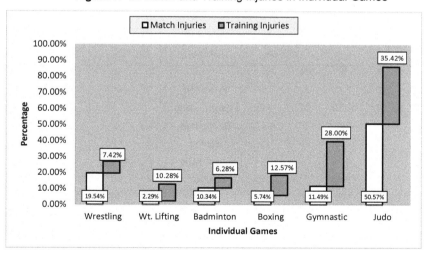

Table IV-46 New and Recurrent Injuries in Team and Individual Games

		N	Percentage
Team Games	New Injuries	217	49.09
	Recurrent Injuries	225	51.01
	Total	**442**	**100**
Individual Games	New Injuries	150	53.38
	Recurrent Injuries	131	46.61
	Total	**281**	**100**

The table 4.46 illustrates the frequencies (N) and percentage distribution of New and Recurrent injuries in Team and Individual Games. In **Team Games** a total 442 new and recurrent were noticed. Out of that 49.09% were new injuries and 51.01% were recurrent injuries. In **Individual Games** total 281 injuries were noticed. Out of the total 53.38% injuries were new and 46.61% injuries were recurrent.

Table IV-47 Game wise Distribution of New and Recurrent Injuries in Team and Individual Games

Team Games	New Injuries		Recurrent Injuries		Individual Games	New Injuries		Training Injuries	
	N	%	N	%		N	%	N	%
Cricket	16	7.37	17	7.55	Wrestling	22	14.66	13	9.92
Baseball	30	13.82	32	14.22	Weight Lifting	17	11.33	7	5.34
Kabaddi	18	8.29	10	4.44	Badminton	12	8	7	5.34
Basketball	30	13.82	36	16	Boxing	32	21.33	32	24.42
Hockey	32	14.74	52	23.11	Gymnastic	19	12.66	38	29
Football	91	41.93	78	34.66	Judo	48	32	34	25.95
Total	**217**	**100**	**225**	**100**	**Total**	**150**	**100**	**131**	**100**

The table 4.47 explores the game wise distribution of new and recurrent injuries in team and individual games. In **Team Games** the percentage distribution of new and recurrent injuries of Cricket were 7.37±7.55, percentage of Baseball were13.82±14.22, in Kabaddi 8.29±4.44, in Basketball 13.22±16, in Hockey 14.74±23.11, in Football 41.93±34.66

respectively. In **Individual Games** percentage distribution of new and recurrent injuries of wrestling were14.66±9.92, in Weight Lifting 11.33±5.34, in Badminton 8±5.34, in Boxing 21.33±24.42, in Gymnastic 12.66±29 and percentage distribution of match and training injuries in Judo were 32±25.95 respectively.

Figure IV-64 Graphical Representation of New and Recurrent Injuries in Team and Individual Games

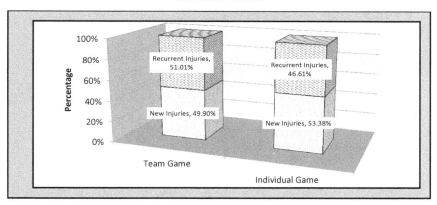

Figure IV-65 Graphical Representation of New and Recurrent Injuries in Team Games

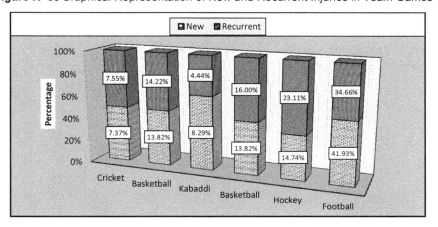

Figure IV-66 Graphical Representation of New and Recurrent Injuries in Individual Games

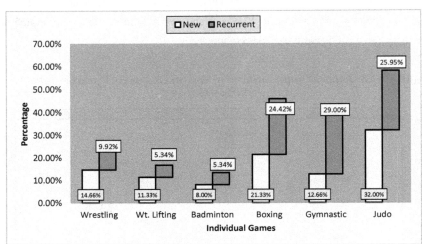

IV.6 Classification of Soft Tissue, Bone and Joint Injuries

Table IV-48 Percentage Distribution of Soft tissue, Bone and Joint Injuries in Team and Individual Games

Team Games	Soft		Bone		Joint		Individual Games	Soft		Bone		Joint	
	N	%	N	%	N	%		N	%	N	%	N	%
Cricket	24	7.10	5	13.51	4	7.01	Wrestling	23	13.37	10	14.08	16	26.66
Baseball	51	15.08	3	8.10	10	17.54	Wt. lifting	18	10.46	0	0	5	8.33
Kabaddi	22	6.50	7	18.91	8	14.03	Badminton	17	9.88	2	2.81	3	5
Basketball	25	7.39	10	27.02	6	10.52	Boxing	16	9.30	41	57.74	4	6.66
Hockey	77	22.78	4	10.81	6	10.52	Gymnastic	37	21.51	12	16.90	10	16.66
football	139	41.12	8	21.62	23	40.35	judo	61	35.46	6	8.45	22	36.66
Total	338	100	37	100	57	100	Total	172	100	71	100	60	100

*N Denotes Frequency

Classification of Soft Tissue, Bone and Joint injuries Team and Individual Game were illustrated in table 4.48 given above. **Team Games:** It was retraced that in Cricket, percentage distribution of soft tissue injuries were 7.10%, bone injuries were 13.51% and joint injuries were 7.01%, in Baseball, percentage of soft tissue injuries were 15.08%, bone injuries 8.10%, joint injuries were 17.54%, in Kabaddi, distribution of soft tissue were 6.50%, bone 18.91%, joint 14.03%, in Basketball, distribution of soft tissue injuries were 7.39%, bone 27.02, joint 10.52%, in Hockey, soft tissue 22.78%, bone 10.81% and joint 10.52% and in Football, the distribution of soft tissue injury type were 41.12%, bone 21.62% and joint 40.35% respectively.

Under the section of **Individual Games**, the percentage distribution of soft, bone and joint injuries of Wrestling were as follow: soft tissue (13.37%), bone (14.08%), Joint (28.66%), in Weight Lifting, soft tissue (10.46%), bone (0), joint (8.33%), in Badminton classification of soft tissue were (9.88%), bone (2.81%), joint (5%), in Boxing percentage distribution of soft tissue injuries were (9.30%), bone (57.74%), joint (6.66%), in Gymnastic classification of soft tissue injuries were (21.51%), bone (16.90%), joint (16.66%), and in Judo the percentage distribution of soft tissue injuries were (35.46%), percentage of joint injuries were (8.45%) and Joint injuries were classified as 35.66% respectively.

Figure IV-67 Graphical Representation of Distribution of Soft tissue, bone and joint injuries in Team Game

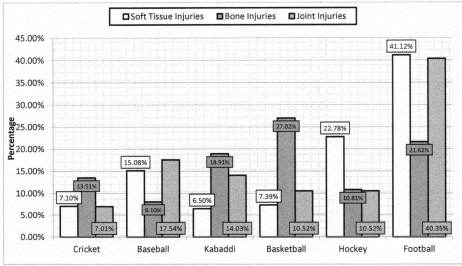

Figure IV-68 Graphical Representation of Distribution of Soft tissue, bone and joint injuries in Individual Games

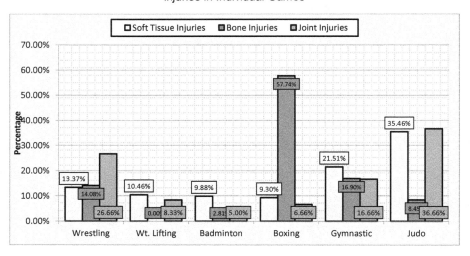

IV.7 Classification of Surface Related Injuries

Table IV-49 Classification of Different Surface Related to Injuries in Team and Individual Games

Surfaces	Team games		Individual games	
	N	%	N	%
Clay	137	36.43	26	14.52
Wooden	2	0.53	0	0
Cemented	22	5.85	1	0.55
Synthetic	83	22.07	43	24.02
Grass	110	29.25	2	1.11
Mat	22	5.85	107	59.77
Total	**376**		**179**	

Table 4.49 classified the surface related injuries of Team and Individual games in the terms of frequencies and percentage. **Team Games:** Accordingly, 137 injuries were reported from clay which constitutes 36.43% of the total injuries, 2 injuries were reported from wooden surface which constitute 0.53% of the total injuries, 22 injuries were reported from Cemented surface which constitute 5.85% of the total injuries, 83 injuries were reported from Synthetic surface which constitute 22.07% of the total injuries, 110 injuries were reported from Grass surface which constitute 29.25% of the total injuries and 22 injuries were reported from mat surface in Team Games which constitute 5.85% of the total injuries. **Individual Games:** 26 injuries were reported from clay which constitutes 14.52% of the total injuries, no injuries were reported from wooden surface in individual games. 1 injury was reported from cemented surface which constitute 0.55% of the total surface, 43 injuries were reported from synthetic surface which constitute 24.02% of the total injuries, 2 injuries were reported from grass surface which constitute 1.11% and 107 injuries were reported on mat surfaces in individual games which constitute 59.77% of the total injuries. It was observed that in team games clay surface are highly probable to injuries and mats are also higher frequency of injuries in individual games.

Figure IV-69 Graphical Representation of Surface Related to Injuries in Team and Individual Games

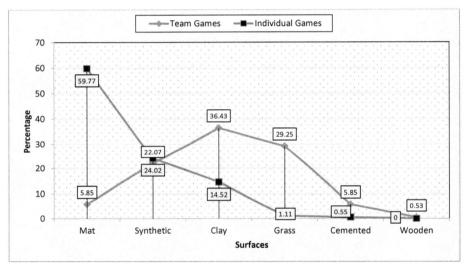

IV.8 Reason of Injuries

IV.8.1 Intrinsic Reasons in Team and Individual Games

Table IV-50 Frequencies and Percentage Distribution of Intrinsic Reason of Injuries in Team Games

		Responses		Percent of
		N	Percent	Cases (IR)
Injury Reasons	Improper Training	17	4.9%	12.5%
	Mentally Disturb	20	5.8%	14.7%
	Over Stretching	23	6.6%	16.9%
	Diet	25	7.2%	18.4%
	Fatigue/Stress	26	7.5%	19.1%
	Fitness	28	8.1%	20.6%
	Over Loading	31	9.0%	22.8%
	Over Training	31	9.0%	22.8%
	Jerk	41	11.8%	30.1%
	Twist	46	13.3%	33.8%
	Improper Warm-up	58	16.8%	42.6%
	Total	**346**	**100.0%**	**254.4%**

Table 4.50 shows the intrinsic reason of injuries in Team Games in the terms of frequency, percentage and percentage of cases (IR). Accordingly, 17 responses are of improper training which constitutes 4.9% and IR 12.5% of the total responses, 20 responses are of mentally disturb which constitute of 5.8% and IR 14.7% of the total responses, 23 responses are of overstretching which constitute 6.6% and IR 16.9% of the total responses, 25 response are relate to diet which constitute 7.2% and IR 18.4% of the total responses, 26 responses are of fatigue/stress which constitute 7.5% and IR 19.1% of the total responses, 28 responses are of fitness which constitute 8.1% and IR 20.6% of the total samples, 31 responses are of over loading and over training which constitute 9.0% and IR 22.8% of the total responses, 41 responses are of jerk which constitute of 11.8% and IR 30.1% of the total sample, 46 responses are of twist which

constitute 13.3% and IR 33.8% of the total sample and 58 responses are of improper warm up which constitute 16.8% and IR 42.6% of the total responses.

Table IV-51 Frequencies and Percentage Distribution of Intrinsic Reason of Injuries in Individual Games

		Responses		Percent of
		N	Percent	Cases
	Improper Training	2	1.0%	2.0%
	Mentally Disturb	3	1.5%	3.0%
	Over Training	11	5.6%	10.9%
	Fatigue/Stress	13	6.6%	12.9%
Injury Reasons	Diet	14	7.1%	13.9%
	Over Loading	16	8.2%	15.8%
	Over Stretching	16	8.2%	15.8%
	Fitness	18	9.2%	17.8%
	Unknown	22	11.2%	21.8%
	Improper Warm-up	23	11.7%	22.8%
	Jerk	28	14.3%	27.7%
	Twist	30	15.3%	29.7%
Total		**196**	**100.0%**	**194.1%**

Table 4.51 shows the intrinsic reasons of sports injuries in Individual Games within the terms of frequencies, percentage and percentage of cases (IR). Accordingly, 2 responses are of improper training which constitute 1% and IR 2% of the total responses, 3 responses are of mentally disturb which constitute 1.5% and IR 3% of the total samples, 11 responses are of overtraining which constitute 5.6% and IR 10.9% of the total sample, 13 responses are of fatigue/stress which constitute 6.6% and IR 12.9% of the total sample, 14 responses are of diet which constitute 7.1% and IR 13.9% of the total sample, 16 responses are of overloading and overstretching which constitute 8.2% and IR 15.8% of the total responses.18 responses are of fitness which constitute 9.2% and IR 17.8% of the total sample. 22 responses are unknown which make 11.2% and IR 21.8% of the total responses. 23 responses are of improper warm-up which makes 11.7% and IR 22.8% of the total responses. 28 responses are of jerk which constitutes 14.3% and IR 27.7% of the total responses. 30 responses are of twist which constitute 15.3% and IR 29.7% of the total responses.

Table IV-52 Intrinsic Cause of Injuries in Cricket

		Responses		Percent of
		N	Percent	Cases
	Diet	3	7.1%	15.0%
	Fatigue/Stress	8	19.0%	40.0%
	Fitness	2	4.8%	10.0%
	Twist	1	2.4%	5.0%
Injury Reasons[b]	Improper warming-up	7	16.7%	35.0%
	Jerk	5	11.9%	25.0%
	Mentally Disturb	2	4.8%	10.0%
	Over Loading	4	9.5%	20.0%
	Over Stretching	2	4.8%	10.0%
	Improper Training	8	19.0%	40.0%
Total		**42**	**100.0%**	**210.0%**

a. Sports = Cricket
b. Dichotomy group tabulated at value 1.

Table 4.52 shows the intrinsic reasons of sports injuries in Cricket within the terms of frequencies, percentage and percentage of cases (IR). Accordingly, 3 responses are of **Diet** which constitute 7.1% and IR 15% of the total responses, 8 responses are of **Fatigue/stress** which constitute 19% and IR 40% of the total samples, 2 responses are of **Fitness** which constitute 4.8% and IR 10% of the total sample, 1 responses are of **Twist** which constitute 2.4% and IR 5% of the total sample, 7 responses are of **Improper warm-up** which constitute 16.7% and IR 35% of the total sample, 5 responses are of **Jerk** which constitute 11.9% and IR 25% of the total responses.2 responses are of **Mentally Disturb** which constitute 4.8% and IR 10% of the total sample. 4 responses are **Overloading** which make 9.5% and IR 20% of the total responses. 2 responses are of **Overstretching** which makes 4.8% and IR 10% of the total responses. 8 responses are of **Improper Training** which constitutes 19% and IR 40% of the total responses.

Table IV-53 Intrinsic Cause of Injuries in Baseball

		Responses		Percent of Cases
		N	Percent	
	Improper Training	2	2.2%	6.5%
	Fatigue/Stress	3	3.2%	9.7%
	Mentally Disturb	5	5.4%	16.1%
	Over Loading	7	7.5%	22.6%
	Over Stretching	8	8.6%	25.8%
Injury Reasons[b]	Jerk	9	9.7%	29.0%
	Fitness	10	10.8%	32.3%
	Twist	10	10.8%	32.3%
	Diet	11	11.8%	35.5%
	Improper warming-up	14	15.1%	45.2%
	Over Training	14	15.1%	45.2%
Total		**93**	**100.0%**	**300.0%**

a. Sports = Baseball
b. Dichotomy group tabulated at value 1.

Table 4.53 shows the intrinsic reasons of sports injuries in Baseball within the terms of frequencies, percentage and percentage of cases (IR). Accordingly, 2 responses are of **Improper Training** which constitute 2.2% and IR 6.5% of the total responses, 3 responses are of **Fatigue/stress** which constitute 3.2% and IR 9.7% of the total samples, 5 responses are of **Mentally Disturb** which constitute 5.4% and IR 16.1% of the total sample, 7 responses are of **Over Loading** which constitute 7.5% and IR 22.6% of the total sample, 8 responses are of **Overstretching** which constitute 8.6% and IR 25.8% of the total sample, 9 responses are of **Jerk** which constitute 9.7%% and IR 29% of the total responses. 10 responses are of **Fitness and Twist** which constitute 10.8% and IR 32.3% of the total sample. 11 responses are **Diet** which make 11.8% and IR 35.5% of the total responses. 14 responses are of **Improper warming-up** and **Over Training** which makes 15.1% and IR 45.2% of the total responses.

Table IV-54 Intrinsic Cause of Injuries in Kabaddi

			Responses		Percent of
			N	Percent	Cases
Injury Reasons[b]	Improper warming-up		2	5.3%	9.5%
	Fatigue/Stress		3	7.9%	14.3%
	Over Training		4	10.5%	19.0%
	Improper Training		4	10.5%	19.0%
	Over Loading		5	13.2%	23.8%
	Twist		6	15.8%	28.6%
	Over Stretching		6	15.8%	28.6%
	Jerk		8	21.1%	38.1%
		Total	**38**	**100.0%**	**181.0%**

a. Sports = Kabaddi
b. Dichotomy group tabulated at value 1.

Table 4.54 shows the intrinsic reasons of sports injuries in Kabaddi within the terms of frequencies, percentage and percentage of cases (IR). Accordingly, 2 responses are of **Improper warming-up** which constitute 5.3% and IR 9.5% of the total responses, 3 responses are of **Fatigue/stress** which constitute 7.9% and IR 14.3% of the total samples, 4 responses are of **Over Training** and **Improper Training** which constitute 10.5% and IR 19% of the total sample, 6 responses are of **Twist** and **Overstretching** which constitute 15.8% and IR 28.6% of the total sample, 8 responses are of **Jerk** which constitute 21.1% and IR 38.1% of the total sample.

Table IV-55 Intrinsic Cause of Injuries in Basketball

		Responses		Percent of Cases
		N	Percent	
	Over Stretching	1	2.0%	4.3%
	Fatigue/Stress	2	4.1%	8.7%
	Mentally Disturb	2	4.1%	8.7%
	Improper Training	2	4.1%	8.7%
Injury Reasons[b]	Diet	3	6.1%	13.0%
	Over Loading	3	6.1%	13.0%
	Over Training	4	8.2%	17.4%
	Jerk	5	10.2%	21.7%
	Fitness	6	12.2%	26.1%
	Twist	10	20.4%	43.5%
	Improper warming-up	11	22.4%	47.8%
Total		**49**	**100.0%**	**213.0%**

a. Sports = Basketball
b. Dichotomy group tabulated at value 1.

Table 4.55 shows the intrinsic reasons of sports injuries in Basketball within the terms of frequencies, percentage and percentage of cases (IR). Accordingly, 1 responses are of **Over Stretching** which constitute 2% and IR 4.3% of the total responses, 2 responses are of **Fatigue/stress, Mentally Disturb and Improper Training** which constitute 4.1% and IR 8.7% of the total samples, 3 responses are of **Diet and Overloading** which constitute 6.1% and IR 13% of the total sample, 4 responses are of **Over Training** which constitute 8.2% and IR 17.4% of the total sample, 5 responses are of **Jerk** which constitute 10.2% and IR 21.7% of the total sample, 6 responses are of **Fitness** which constitute 12.2%% and IR 26.1% of the total responses.10 responses are of **Twist** which constitute 20.4% and IR 43.5% of the total sample.11 responses are **Improper Warming-up** which make 22.4% and IR 47.8% of the total responses.

Table IV-56 Intrinsic Cause of Injuries in Hockey

| | | Responses | | Percent of |
		N	Percent	Cases
	Over Stretching	1	2.7%	7.7%
	Over Training	1	2.7%	7.7%
	Fatigue/Stress	2	5.4%	15.4%
	Mentally Disturb	2	5.4%	15.4%
Injury Reasons[b]	Fitness	3	8.1%	23.1%
	Diet	4	10.8%	30.8%
	Jerk	5	13.5%	38.5%
	Over Loading	5	13.5%	38.5%
	Improper warming-up	6	16.2%	46.2%
	Twist	8	21.6%	61.5%
Total		37	100.0%	284.6%

a. Sports = Hockey
b. Dichotomy group tabulated at value 1.

Table 4.56 shows the intrinsic reasons of sports injuries in Hockey within the terms of frequencies, percentage and percentage of cases (IR). Accordingly,1 responses are of **Over Stretching and Over Training** which constitute 2.7% and IR 7.7% of the total responses, 2 responses are of **Fatigue/stress** and **Mentally Disturb** which constitute 5.4% and IR 15.4% of the total samples, 3 responses are of **Fitness** which constitute 8.1% and IR 23.1% of the total sample, 4 responses are of **Diet** which constitute 10.8% and IR 30.8% of the total sample, 5 responses are of **Jerk and Overloading** which constitute 13.5% and IR 38.5% of the total sample, 6 responses are of **Improper Warming-Up** which constitute 16.2% and IR 46.2% of the total responses.8 responses are of **Twist** which constitute 21.6% and IR 61.5% of the total sample.

Table IV-57 Intrinsic Cause of Injuries in Football

		Responses		Percent of
		N	Percent	Cases
Injury Reasons[b]	Improper Training	1	1.1%	3.6%
	Diet	4	4.6%	14.3%
	Over Stretching	5	5.7%	17.9%
	Fitness	7	8.0%	25.0%
	Over Loading	7	8.0%	25.0%
	Fatigue/Stress	8	9.2%	28.6%
	Over Training	8	9.2%	28.6%
	Jerk	9	10.3%	32.1%
	Mentally Disturb	9	10.3%	32.1%
	Twist	11	12.6%	39.3%
	Improper warming-up	18	20.7%	64.3%
Total		**87**	**100.0%**	**310.7%**

a. Sports = Football
b. Dichotomy group tabulated at value 1.

Table 4.57 shows the intrinsic reasons of sports injuries in Football within the terms of frequencies, percentage and percentage of cases (IR). Accordingly,1 responses are of **Improper Training** which constitute 1.1% and IR 3.6% of the total responses, 4 responses are of **Diet** which constitute 4.6% and IR 14.3% of the total samples, 5 responses are of **Over Stretching** which constitute 5.7% and IR 17.9% of the total sample, 7 responses are of **Fitness** and **Overloading** which constitute 8% and IR 25% of the total sample, 8 responses are of **Fatigue/stress and Over Training** which constitute 9.2% and IR 28.6% of the total sample, 9 responses are of **Jerk and Mentally Disturb** which constitute 10.3%% and IR 32.1% of the total responses.11 responses are of **Twist** which constitute 12.6% and IR 39.3% of the total sample.18 responses are **Improper Warming-up** which make 20.7% and IR 64.3% of the total responses.

Figure IV-70 Graphical Representation of Distribution of Intrinsic Causes of Injuries in Team Games

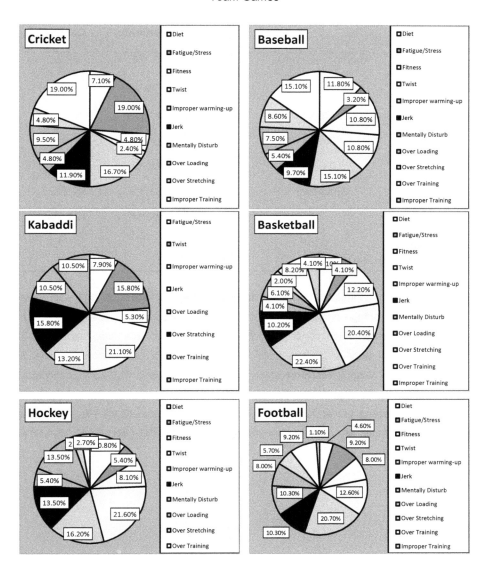

Table IV-58 Intrinsic Cause of Injuries in Wrestling

		Responses		Percent of
		N	Percent	Cases
Individual	Improper Warm-up	1	3.7%	4.8%
Games[b]	Jerk	2	7.4%	9.5%
	Over Stretching	3	11.1%	14.3%
	Fitness	4	14.8%	19.0%
	Twist	8	29.6%	38.1%
	Unknown	9	33.3%	42.9%
Total		**27**	**100.0%**	**128.6%**

a. Sports = Wrestling
b. Dichotomy group tabulated at value 1.

Table 4.58 shows the intrinsic reasons of sports injuries in **Wrestling** within the terms of frequencies, percentage and percentage of cases (IR). Accordingly,1 responses are of **Improper Warm-up** which constitute 3.7% and IR 4.8% of the total responses, 2 responses are of **Jerk** which constitute 7.4% and IR 9.5% of the total samples, 3 responses are of **Over Stretching** which constitute 11.1% and IR 14.3% of the total sample, 4 responses are of **Fitness** which constitute 14.8% and IR 19% of the total sample, 8 responses are of **Twist** which constitute 29.6% and IR 38.1% of the total sample, 9 responses are of **Unknown** which constitute 33.3%% and IR 42.9% of the total responses.

Table IV-59 Intrinsic Cause of Injuries in Weight Lifting

		Responses		Percent of
		N	Percent	Cases
Individual	Over Stretching	1	4.8%	7.1%
Games[b]	Diet	2	9.5%	14.3%
	Fitness	2	9.5%	14.3%
	Twist	2	9.5%	14.3%
	Fatigue/Stress	3	14.3%	21.4%
	Improper Warm-up	3	14.3%	21.4%
	Jerk	3	14.3%	21.4%
	Over Loading	5	23.8%	35.7%
	Total	**21**	**100.0%**	**150.0%**

a. Sports = Weight Lifting

b. Dichotomy group tabulated at value 1.

Table 4.59 shows the intrinsic reasons of sports injuries in **Weight Lifting** within the terms of frequencies, percentage and percentage of cases (IR). Accordingly,1 responses are of **Over Stretching** which constitute 4.8% and IR 7.1% of the total responses, 2 responses are of **Diet, Fitness** and **Twist** which constitute 9.5% and IR 14.3% of the total samples, 3 responses are of **Fatigue/Stress, Improper Warming-up and Jerk** which constitute14.3% and IR 21.4% of the total sample, 5 responses are of **Overloading** which constitute 23.8% and IR 35.7% of the total sample.

Table IV-60 Intrinsic Cause of Injuries in Badminton

		Responses		Percent of
		N	Percent	Cases
Individual Games[b]	Over Loading	1	2.6%	5.9%
	Diet	2	5.1%	11.8%
	Fatigue/Stress	2	5.1%	11.8%
	Over Training	2	5.1%	11.8%
	Improper Training	2	5.1%	11.8%
	Unknown	3	7.7%	17.6%
	Twist	4	10.3%	23.5%
	Improper Warm-up	6	15.4%	35.3%
	Over Stretching	6	15.4%	35.3%
	Jerk	11	28.2%	64.7%
Total		**39**	**100.0%**	**229.4%**

a. Sports = Badminton
b. Dichotomy group tabulated at value 1.

Table 4.60 shows the intrinsic reasons of sports injuries in **Badminton** within the terms of frequencies, percentage and percentage of cases (IR). Accordingly,1 responses are of **Over Loading** which constitute 2.6% and IR 5.9% of the total responses, 2 responses are of **Fatigue/stress, Overtraining, Improper Training and Diet** which constitute 5.1% and IR 11.8% of the total samples, 3 responses are of **Unknown** which constitute 7.7% and IR 17.6% of the total sample, 4 responses are of **Twist** which constitute 10.3% and IR 23.5% of the total sample, 6 responses are of **Improper warm-up and Overstretching** which constitute 15.4% and IR 35.3% of the total sample,11 responses are of **Jerk** which constitute 28.2%% and IR 64.7% of the total responses.

Table IV-61 Intrinsic Cause of Injuries in Boxing

| | | Responses | | Percent of |
		N	Percent	Cases
Individual	Fitness	2	8.3%	9.5%
Games[b]	Improper Warm-up	3	12.5%	14.3%
	Jerk	3	12.5%	14.3%
	Over Loading	4	16.7%	19.0%
	Over Training	5	20.8%	23.8%
	Unknown	7	29.2%	33.3%
Total		**24**	**100.0%**	**114.3%**

a. Sports = Boxing

b. Dichotomy group tabulated at value 1.

Table 4.61 shows the intrinsic reasons of sports injuries in **Boxing** within the terms of frequencies, percentage and percentage of cases (IR). Accordingly,2 responses are of **Fitness** which constitute 8.3% and IR 9.5% of the total responses, 3 responses are of **Improper Warm-up** and **Jerk** which constitute 12.5% and IR 14.3% of the total samples, 4 responses are of **Over Loading** which constitute 16.7% and IR 19% of the total sample,5 responses are of **Over Training** which constitute 20.8% and IR 23.8% of the total sample, 7 responses are of **Unknown** which constitute 29.2% and IR 33.3% of the total responses.

Table IV-62 Intrinsic Cause of Injuries in Gymnastic

		Responses		Percent of
		N	Percent	Cases
Individual	Mentally Disturb	2	3.7%	11.1%
Games[b]	Over Training	2	3.7%	11.1%
	Over Stretching	3	5.6%	16.7%
	Unknown	3	5.6%	16.7%
	Fatigue/Stress	4	7.4%	22.2%
	Over Loading	4	7.4%	22.2%
	Improper Warm-up	5	9.3%	27.8%
	Diet	6	11.1%	33.3%
	Fitness	7	13.0%	38.9%
	Jerk	8	14.8%	44.4%
	Twist	10	18.5%	55.6%
Total		**54**	**100.0%**	**300.0%**

a. Sports = Gymnastic
b. Dichotomy group tabulated at value 1.

Table 4.62 shows the intrinsic reasons of sports injuries in **Gymnastic** within the terms of frequencies, percentage and percentage of cases (IR). Accordingly,2 responses are of **Mentally Disturb** and **Over Training** which constitute 3.7% and IR 11.1% of the total responses, 3 responses are of **Overstretching** and **Unknown** which constitute 5.6% and IR 16.7% of the total samples, 4 responses are of **Fatigue/stress and Overloading** which constitute 7.4% and IR 22.2% of the total sample, 5 responses are of **Improper Warm-up** which constitute 9.3% and IR 27.8% of the total sample, 6 responses are of **Diet** which constitute 11.1% and IR 33.3% of the total sample, 7 responses are of **Fitness** which constitute 13%% and IR 38.9% of the total responses.8 responses are of **Jerk** which constitute 14.8% and IR 44.4% of the total sample.10 responses are **Twist** which make 18.5% and IR 55.6% of the total responses.

Table IV-63 Intrinsic Cause of Injuries in Judo

		Responses		Percent of
		N	Percent	Cases
Individual	Jerk	1	3.3%	11.1%
Games[b]	Mentally Disturb	1	3.3%	11.1%
	Over Loading	2	6.7%	22.2%
	Over Training	2	6.7%	22.2%
	Fitness	3	10.0%	33.3%
	Over Stretching	3	10.0%	33.3%
	Diet	4	13.3%	44.4%
	Fatigue/Stress	4	13.3%	44.4%
	Twist	5	16.7%	55.6%
	Improper Warm-up	5	16.7%	55.6%
Total		**30**	**100.0%**	**333.3%**

a. Sports = Judo
b. Dichotomy group tabulated at value 1.

Table 4.63 shows the intrinsic reasons of sports injuries in **Judo** within the terms of frequencies, percentage and percentage of cases (IR). Accordingly,1 response is of **Jerk** and **Mentally Disturb** which constitute 3.3% and IR 11.1% of the total responses, 2 responses are of **Over Loading** and **Overtraining** which constitute 6.7% and IR 22.2% of the total samples, 3 responses are of **Fitness and Overstretching** which constitute 10% and IR 33.3% of the total sample, 4 responses are of **Diet and Fatigue/Stress** which constitute 13.3% and IR 44.4% of the total sample, 5 responses are of **Twist** and **Improper Warm-up** which constitute 16.7% and IR 55.6% of the total responses.

Figure IV-71 Graphical Representation of Distribution of Intrinsic Causes of Injuries in Individual Games

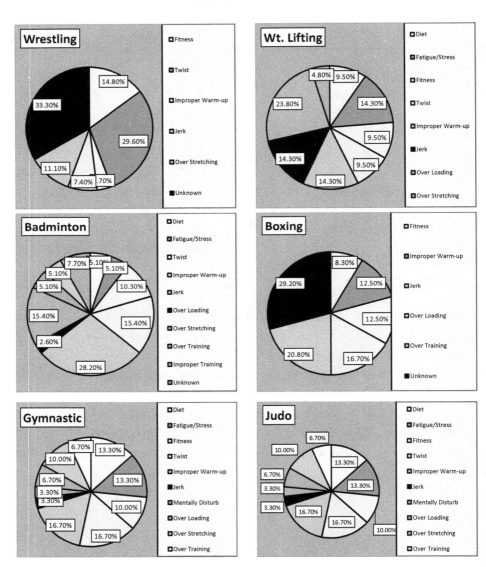

IV.8.2 Extrinsic Reasons in Team and Individual Games

Table IV-64 Frequencies and Percentage Distribution of Extrinsic Reason of Injuries in Team Games

		Responses		Percent of Cases
		N	Percent	
Team Game	Bare Foot	9	3.2%	6.6%
	Climatic Condition	12	4.3%	8.8%
	Faulty Equipment	14	5.0%	10.3%
	Kit/Footwear	16	5.7%	11.8%
	Playing Environment	21	7.5%	15.4%
	Poor Technique	27	9.7%	19.9%
	Collision Impact	28	10.0%	20.6%
	Unknown	30	10.8%	22.1%
	Carelessness	32	11.5%	23.5%
	Fall or Slip	43	15.4%	31.6%
	Field/Playground	47	16.8%	34.6%
Total		**279**	**100.0%**	**205.1%**

a. Game Type = Team Game
b. Dichotomy group tabulated at value 1.

Table 4.64 shows the extrinsic reasons of sports injuries in **Team Games** within the terms of frequencies, percentage and percentage of cases (IR). Accordingly,9 responses are of **Bare Foot** which constitute 3.2% and IR 6.6% of the total responses, 12 responses are of **Climatic Condition** which constitute 4.3% and IR 8.8% of the total samples, 14 responses are of **Faulty Equipment** which constitute 5% and IR 10.3% of the total sample, 16 responses are of **Kit/Footwear** which constitute 5.7% and IR 11.8% of the total sample, 21 responses are of **Playing Environment** which constitute 7.5% and IR 15.4% of the total sample, 27 responses are of **Poor Technique** which constitute 9.7%% and IR 19.9% of the total responses. 28 responses are of **Collision Impact** which constitute 10% and IR 20.6% of the total sample.30 responses are **Unknown** which make 10.8% and IR 22.1% of the total responses. 32 responses are of **Carelessness** which constitute 11.5% and IR 23.5% of the total responses. 43

responses are of Fall or Slip which constitute 15.4% and IR 31.6% of the total responses and 47 responses are of Field/Playground which constitute 16.8% and IR 34.6% of the total responses.

Table IV-65 Frequencies and Percentage Distribution of Extrinsic Reason of Injuries in Individual Games

		Responses		Percent of Cases
		N	Percent	
-b	Bare Foot	3	1.9%	3.0%
	Climatic Condition	4	2.5%	4.0%
	Playing Environment	5	3.1%	5.0%
	Faulty Equipment	8	5.0%	7.9%
	Carelessness	11	6.9%	10.9%
	Kit/Footwear	11	6.9%	10.9%
	Field/Playground	13	8.2%	12.9%
	Poor Technique	19	11.9%	18.8%
	Unknown	21	13.2%	20.8%
	Fall or Slip	28	17.6%	27.7%
	Collision Impact	36	22.6%	35.6%
Total		**159**	**100.0%**	**157.4%**

a. Game Type = Individual Game
b. Dichotomy group tabulated at value 1.

Table 4.65 shows the extrinsic reasons of sports injuries in **Individual Games** within the terms of frequencies, percentage and percentage of cases (IR). Accordingly,3 responses are of **Bare Foot** which constitute 1.9% and IR 3% of the total responses, 4 responses are of **Climatic Condition** which constitute 2.5% and IR 4% of the total samples, 5 responses are of **Playing Environment** which constitute 3.1% and IR 5% of the total sample, 8 responses are of **Faulty Equipment** which constitute 5% and IR 7.9% of the total sample, 11 responses are of **Carelessness and Kit/Footwear** which constitute 6.9% and IR 10.9% of the total sample,13 responses are of **Field /Playground** which constitute 8.2%% and IR 12.9% of the total responses. 19 responses are of **Poor Technique** which constitute 11.9% and IR 18.8% of the total sample.21 responses are **Unknown** which make 13.2% and IR 20.8% of the total responses. 28 responses are of **Fall or slip** which constitute 17.6% and IR 27.7% of the total responses. 36 responses are of Collision Impact which constitute 22.6%% and IR 35.6% of the total responses.

Table IV-66 Extrinsic Reasons of Injuries in Cricket

		Responses		Percent of
		N	Percent	Cases
Reasons[b]	Climatic Condition	2	8.0%	11.1%
	Collision Impact	2	8.0%	11.1%
	Poor Technique	2	8.0%	11.1%
	Carelessness	3	12.0%	16.7%
	Fall or Slip	3	12.0%	16.7%
	Field/Playground	4	16.0%	22.2%
	Kit/Footwear	4	16.0%	22.2%
	Unknown	5	20.0%	27.8%
Total		25	100.0%	138.9%

a. Sports = CRICKET
b. Dichotomy group tabulated at value 1.

Table 4.66 shows the extrinsic reasons of sports injuries in **Cricket** within the terms of frequencies, percentage and percentage of cases (IR). Accordingly,2 responses are of **Climatic Condition, Collision/Impact and Poor Technique** which constitute 8% and IR 11.1% of the total responses, 3 responses are of **Carelessness and Fall or Slip** which constitute 12% and IR 16.7% of the total samples, 4 responses are of **Field/Playground and Kit/Footwear** which constitute 16% and IR 22.2% of the total sample, 5 responses are **Unknown** which constitute 20% and IR 27.8% of the total responses.

Table IV-67 Extrinsic Reasons of Injuries in Baseball

		Responses		Percent of
		N	Percent	Cases
Reasons[b]	Climatic Condition	1	1.6%	3.1%
	Bare Foot	2	3.2%	6.2%
	Kit/Footwear	3	4.8%	9.4%
	Collision Impact	4	6.3%	12.5%
	Faulty Equipment	4	6.3%	12.5%
	Playing Environment	6	9.5%	18.8%
	Unknown	7	11.1%	21.9%
	Fall or Slip	8	12.7%	25.0%
	Carelessness	9	14.3%	28.1%
	Field/Playground	9	14.3%	28.1%
	Poor Technique	10	15.9%	31.2%
Total		**63**	**100.0%**	**196.9%**

a. Sports = BASEBALL
b. Dichotomy group tabulated at value 1.

Table 4.67 shows the extrinsic reasons of sports injuries in **Baseball** within the terms of frequencies, percentage and percentage of cases (IR). Accordingly,1 response is of **Climatic Condition** which constitute 1.6% and IR 3.1% of the total responses, 2 responses are of **Bare Foot** which constitute 3.2% and IR 6.2% of the total samples, 3 responses are of **Kit/Footwear** which constitute 4.8% and IR 9.4% of the total sample, 4 responses are of **Collision/Impact** and **Faulty Equipment** which constitute 6.3% and IR 12.5% of the total sample, 6 responses are of **Playing Environment** which constitute 9.5% and IR 18.8% of the total sample,7 responses are of **Unknown** which constitute 11.1%% and IR 21.9% of the total responses. 8 responses are of **Fall or Slip** which constitute 12.7% and IR 25% of the total sample.9 responses are **Carelessness** **and Field/Playground** which make 14.3% and IR 28.1% of the total responses. 10 responses are of **Poor Technique** which constitute 15.9% and IR 31.2% of the total responses.

Table IV-68 Extrinsic Reasons of Injuries in Kabaddi

		Responses		Percent of Cases
		N	Percent	
Reasons[b]	Climatic Condition	1	2.8%	5.0%
	Poor Technique	1	2.8%	5.0%
	Carelessness	3	8.3%	15.0%
	Unknown	4	11.1%	20.0%
	Bare Foot	5	13.9%	25.0%
	Collision Impact	6	16.7%	30.0%
	Fall or Slip	7	19.4%	35.0%
	Field/Playground	9	25.0%	45.0%
Total		36	100.0%	180.0%

a. Sports = KABADDI
b. Dichotomy group tabulated at value 1.

Table 4.68 shows the extrinsic reasons of sports injuries in **Kabaddi** within the terms of frequencies, percentage and percentage of cases (IR). Accordingly,1 response is of **Climatic Condition** and **Poor Technique** which constitute 2.8% and IR 5% of the total responses, 3 responses are of **Carelessness** which constitute 8.3% and IR 15% of the total samples, 4 responses are of **Unknown** which constitute 11.1% and IR 20% of the total sample, 5 responses are of **Bare Foot** which constitute 13.9% and IR 25% of the total sample, 6 responses are of **Collision/Impact** which constitute 16.7% and IR 30% of the total sample,7 responses are of **Fall or Slip** which constitute 19.4% and IR 35% of the total responses. 9 responses are of **Field/Playground** which constitute 25% and IR 45% of the total responses.

Table IV-69 Extrinsic Reasons of Injuries in Basketball

		Responses		Percent of
		N	Percent	Cases
Reasons[b]	Climatic Condition	1	2.4%	4.5%
	Fall or Slip	2	4.9%	9.1%
	Collision Impact	3	7.3%	13.6%
	Carelessness	4	9.8%	18.2%
	Playing Environment	4	9.8%	18.2%
	Field/Playground	6	14.6%	27.3%
	Poor Technique	7	17.1%	31.8%
	Faulty Equipment	7	17.1%	31.8%
	Unknown	7	17.1%	31.8%
Total		41	100.0%	186.4%

a. Sports = BASKETBALL
b. Dichotomy group tabulated at value 1.

Table 4.69 shows the extrinsic reasons of sports injuries in **Basketball** within the terms of frequencies, percentage and percentage of cases (IR). Accordingly,1 response is of **Climatic Condition** which constitute 2.4% and IR 4.5% of the total responses, 2 responses are of **Fall or Slip** which constitute 4.9% and IR 9.1% of the total samples, 3 responses are of **Collision/Impact** which constitute 7.3% and IR 13.6% of the total sample, 4 responses are of **Carelessness** and **Playing Environment** which constitute 9.8% and IR 18.2% of the total sample, 6 responses are of **Field/Playground** which constitute 14.6% and IR 27.3% of the total sample,7 responses are of **Poor Technique, Faulty Equipment** and **Unknown** which constitute 17.1% and IR 31.8% of the total responses.

Table IV-70 Extrinsic Reasons of Injuries in Hockey

		Responses		Percent of
		N	**Percent**	**Cases**
Reasons[b]	Carelessness	1	5.9%	7.1%
	Kit/Footwear	2	11.8%	14.3%
	Collision Impact	3	17.6%	21.4%
	Unknown	3	17.6%	21.4%
	Fall or Slip	4	23.5%	28.6%
	Field/Playground	4	23.5%	28.6%
Total		**17**	**100.0%**	**121.4%**

a. Sports = HOCKEY
b. Dichotomy group tabulated at value 1.

Table 4.70 shows the extrinsic reasons of sports injuries in **Hockey** players within the terms of frequencies, percentage and percentage of cases (IR). Accordingly, 1 response is of **Carelessness** which constitute 5.9% and IR 7.1% of the total responses, 2 responses are of **Kit/Footwear** which constitute 11.8% and IR 14.3% of the total samples, 3 responses are of **Collision/Impact** and **Unknown** which constitute 17.6% and IR 21.4% of the total sample, 4 responses are of **Fall or Slip and Field/Playground** which constitute 23.5% and IR 28.6% of the total responses.

Table IV-71 Extrinsic Reasons of Injuries in Football

		Responses		Percent of
		N	Percent	Cases
Reasons[b]	Bare Foot	2	2.1%	6.7%
	Faulty Equipment	3	3.1%	10.0%
	Unknown	4	4.1%	13.3%
	Climatic Condition	7	7.2%	23.3%
	Poor Technique	7	7.2%	23.3%
	Kit/Footwear	7	7.2%	23.3%
	Collision Impact	10	10.3%	33.3%
	Playing Environment	11	11.3%	36.7%
	Carelessness	12	12.4%	40.0%
	Field/Playground	15	15.5%	50.0%
	Fall or Slip	19	19.6%	63.3%
Total		97	100.0%	323.3%

a. Sports = FOOTBALL
b. Dichotomy group tabulated at value 1.

Table 4.71 shows the extrinsic reasons of sports injuries in **Football** within the terms of frequencies, percentage and percentage of cases (IR). Accordingly,2 responses are of **Bare Foot** which constitute 2.1% and IR 6.7% of the total responses, 3 responses are of **Faulty Equipment** which constitute 3.1% and IR 10% of the total samples, 4 responses are of **Unknown** which constitute 4.1% and IR 13.3% of the total sample, 7 responses are of **Climatic Condition, Poor Technique and Kit/Footwear** which constitute 7.2% and IR 23.3% of the total sample, 10 responses are of **Collision/Impact0** which constitute 10.3% and IR 33.3% of the total sample,11 responses are of **Playing Environment** which constitute 11.3%% and IR 36.7% of the total responses. 12 responses are of **Carelessness** which constitute 12.4% and IR 40% of the total sample.15 responses are **Field/Playground** which make 15.5% and IR 50% of the total responses. 19 responses are of **Fall or Slip** which constitute 19.6% and IR 63.3% of the total responses.

Table IV-72 Extrinsic Reasons of Injuries in Wrestling

		Responses		Percent of
		N	Percent	Cases
Reasons[b]	Climatic Condition	1	4.2%	4.8%
	Field/Playground	1	4.2%	4.8%
	Fall or Slip	5	20.8%	23.8%
	Unknown	5	20.8%	23.8%
	Collision Impact	12	50.0%	57.1%
Total		24	100.0%	114.3%

a. Sports = WRESTLING
b. Dichotomy group tabulated at value 1.

Table 4.72 shows the extrinsic reasons of sports injuries in **Wrestling** players within the terms of frequencies, percentage and percentage of cases (IR). Accordingly, 1 response is of **Climatic Condition** and **Field/Playground** which constitute 4.2% and IR 4.8% of the total responses, 5 responses are of **Fall or Slip/Unknown** which constitute 20.8% and IR 23.8% of the total samples, 12 responses are of **Collision/Impact** which constitute 50% and IR 57.1% of the total responses.

Table IV-73 Extrinsic Reasons of Injuries in Weight Lifting

		Responses		Percent of
		N	Percent	Cases
Reasons[b]	Kit/Footwear	1	5.6%	7.1%
	Carelessness	2	11.1%	14.3%
	Fall or Slip	2	11.1%	14.3%
	Faulty Equipment	2	11.1%	14.3%
	Unknown	3	16.7%	21.4%
	Poor Technique	8	44.4%	57.1%
Total		18	100.0%	128.6%

a. Sports = WEIGHT LIFITING
b. Dichotomy group tabulated at value 1.

Table 4.73 shows the extrinsic reasons of sports injuries in **Weight Lifting** players within the terms of frequencies, percentage and percentage of cases (IR). Accordingly, 1 response is of **Kit/Footwear** which constitute 5.6% and IR 7.1% of the total responses, 2 responses are of **Carelessness, Fall or Slip** and **Faulty Equipment** which constitute 11.1% and IR 14.3% of the total samples, 3 responses are of **Unknown** which constitute 16.7% and IR 21.4% of the total responses. 8 responses are of **Poor Technique** which makes 44.4% and IR 57.1% of the total sample.

Table IV-74 Extrinsic Reasons of Injuries in Badminton

		Responses		Percent of
		N	Percent	Cases
Reasons[b]	Carelessness	1	4.0%	6.2%
	Collision Impact	1	4.0%	6.2%
	Kit/Footwear	1	4.0%	6.2%
	Poor Technique	2	8.0%	12.5%
	Playing Environment	2	8.0%	12.5%
	Climatic Condition	3	12.0%	18.8%
	Field/Playground	4	16.0%	25.0%
	Unknown	5	20.0%	31.2%
	Fall or Slip	6	24.0%	37.5%
Total		**25**	**100.0%**	**156.2%**

a. Sports = BADMINTON
b. Dichotomy group tabulated at value 1.

Table 4.74 shows the extrinsic reasons of sports injuries in **Badminton** within the terms of frequencies, percentage and percentage of cases (IR). Accordingly,1 responses are of **Carelessness, Collision Impact and Kit/Footwear** which constitute 4% and IR 6.2% of the total responses, 2 responses are of **Poor Technique and Playing Environment** which constitute 8% and IR 12.5% of the total samples, 3 responses are of **Climatic Condition** which constitute 12% and IR 18.8% of the total sample, 4 responses are of **Field/Playground** which constitute 16% and IR 25% of the total sample, 5 responses are of **Unknown** which constitute 20% and IR 31.2% of the total sample,6 responses are of **Fall or Slip** which constitute 24.4%% and IR 37.5% of the total responses.

Table IV-75 Extrinsic Reasons of Injuries in Boxing

		Responses		Percent of Cases
		N	Percent	
Reasons[b]	Kit/Footwear	1	3.1%	4.8%
	Unknown	1	3.1%	4.8%
	Fall or Slip	2	6.2%	9.5%
	Faulty Equipment	2	6.2%	9.5%
	Carelessness	3	9.4%	14.3%
	Poor Technique	5	15.6%	23.8%
	Collision Impact	18	56.2%	85.7%
Total		**32**	**100.0%**	**152.4%**

a. Sports = BOXING
b. Dichotomy group tabulated at value 1.

Table 4.75 shows the extrinsic reasons of sports injuries in **Boxing** within the terms of frequencies, percentage and percentage of cases (IR). Accordingly,1 responses are of **Kit/Footwear** and **Unknown** which constitute 3.1% and IR 4.8% of the total responses, 2 responses are of **Fall or Slip/** and **Faulty Equipment** which constitute 6.2% and IR 9.5% of the total samples, 3 responses are of **Carelessness** which constitute 9.4% and IR 14.3% of the total sample, 5 responses are of **Poor Technique** which constitute 15.6% and IR 23.8% of the total sample, 18 responses are of **Collision/Impact** which constitute 56.2% and IR 85.7% of the total responses.

Table IV-76 Extrinsic Reasons of Injuries in Gymnastic

		Responses		Percent of Cases
		N	Percent	
Reasons[b]	Carelessness	1	2.9%	5.6%
	Playing Environment	1	2.9%	5.6%
	Poor Technique	2	5.9%	11.1%
	Bare Foot	3	8.8%	16.7%
	Faulty Equipment	4	11.8%	22.2%
	Kit/Footwear	4	11.8%	22.2%
	Unknown	4	11.8%	22.2%
	Field/Playground	7	20.6%	38.9%
	Fall or Slip	8	23.5%	44.4%
Total		**34**	**100.0%**	**188.9%**

a. Sports = GYMNASTIC
b. Dichotomy group tabulated at value 1.

Table 4.76 shows the extrinsic reasons of sports injuries in **Gymnastic** within the terms of frequencies, percentage and percentage of cases (IR). Accordingly, 1 responses are of **Carelessness and Playing Environment** which constitute 2.9% and IR 5.6% of the total responses, 2 responses are of **Poor Technique** which constitute 5.9% and IR 11.1% of the total samples, 3 responses are of **Bare Foot** which constitute 8.8% and IR 16.7% of the total sample, 4 responses are of **Faulty Equipment, Kit/Footwear** and **Unknown** which constitute 11.8% and IR 22.2% of the total sample, 7 responses are of **Field/Playground** which constitute 20.6% and IR 38.9% of the total responses. 8 responses are of **Fall or Slip** which makes 23.5% and IR 44.4% of the total sample.

Table IV-77 Extrinsic Reasons of Injuries in Judo

		Responses		Percent of
		N	Percent	Cases
Reasons[b]	Field/Playground	1	3.8%	9.1%
	Poor Technique	2	7.7%	18.2%
	Playing Environment	2	7.7%	18.2%
	Unknown	3	11.5%	27.3%
	Carelessness	4	15.4%	36.4%
	Kit/Footwear	4	15.4%	36.4%
	Collision Impact	5	19.2%	45.5%
	Fall or Slip	5	19.2%	45.5%
Total		**26**	**100.0%**	**236.4%**

a. Sports = JUDO
b. Dichotomy group tabulated at value 1.

Table 4.77 shows the extrinsic reasons of sports injuries in **Judo** within the terms of frequencies, percentage and percentage of cases (IR). Accordingly,1 responses are of **Field/Playground** which constitute 3.8% and IR 9.1% of the total responses, 2 responses are of **Poor Technique** and **Playing Environment** which constitute 7.7% and IR 18.2% of the total samples, 3 responses are of **Unknown** which constitute 11.5% and IR 27.3% of the total responses, 4 responses are of **Carelessness** and **Kit/Footwear** which constitute 15.4% and IR 36.4% of the total sample, 5 responses are of **Collision Impact** and **Fall or Slip** which constitute 19.2% and IR 45.5% of the total responses.

Figure IV-72 Graphical Representation of Distribution of Extrinsic Causes of Injuries in Team Game

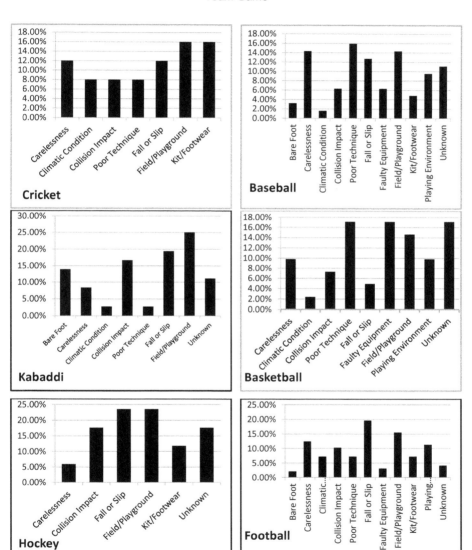

Figure IV-73 Graphical Representation of Distribution of Extrinsic Causes of Injuries in Individual Game

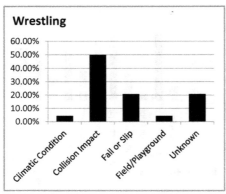

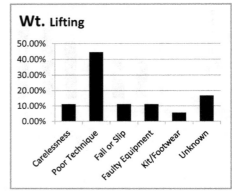

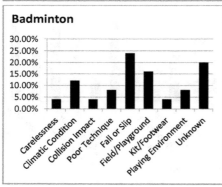

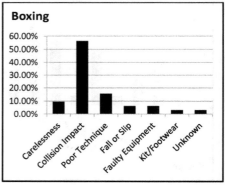

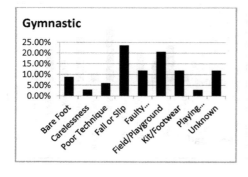

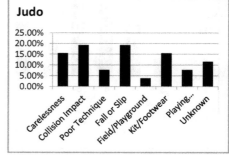

IV.9 Comparison of Frequencies Distribution between Team and Individual Sports in Relation to Sports Injuries.

Table IV-78 Cross Tabulation of Frequencies of Abrasion between Team and Individual Game

			GAME TYPE		Total
			Team Game	Individual Game	
Abrasion	Not Injured	Count	69	114	183
		Expected Count	92.7	90.3	183.0
	Injured	Count	83	34	117
		Expected Count	59.3	57.7	117.0
Total		Count	152	148	300
		Expected Count	152.0	148.0	300.0

Figure IV-74 Distribution of Frequencies of Abrasion between Team and Individual Games

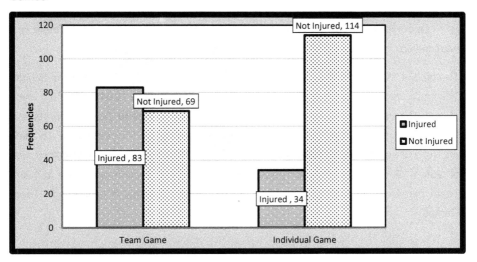

Table IV-79 Comparison between Observed and Expected Frequencies of Abrasion

	Value	df	Asymp. Sig. (2-sided)	Exact Sig. (2-sided)	Exact Sig. (1-sided)
			Chi-Square Tests		
Pearson Chi-Square	31.539[a]	1	.000		
Continuity Correction[b]	30.224	1	.000		
Likelihood Ratio	32.294	1	.000		
Fisher's Exact Test				.000	.000
Linear-by-Linear Association	31.434	1	.000		
N of Valid Cases	300				

a. 0 cells (0.0%) have expected count less than 5. The minimum expected count is 57.72.
b. Computed only for a 2x2 table

$H1_0$= **Occurrence of Abrasion and type of sports are independent** - there is no relationship.

$H1_1$= **Occurrence of Abrasion and type of sports are not independent** - there is a relationship.

The table 4.79 revealed that the association between Abrasion and Game Type is high. The calculated value of χ^2 (31.539) is more than the table value (3.84) at $P \leq 0.5$ level, df =1. The null hypothesis (H_0) "Occurrence of Abrasion and type of sports are independent" thus, is rejected while alternative hypothesis (H_1) "Occurrence of Abrasion and type of sports are not independent" is accepted. This is evident from the illustration of table 4.78 where the highest frequencies of injured respondents are come from the Team games. It means the probability of occurrence of Abrasion is higher in Team Games.

Table IV-80 Cross Tabulation of Frequencies of Blisters between Team and Individual Game

			GAME TYPE		Total
		Crosstab	Team Game	Individual Game	
Blisters	Not Injured	Count	123	125	248
		Expected Count	125.7	122.3	248.0
	Injured	Count	29	23	52
		Expected Count	26.3	25.7	52.0
Total		Count	152	148	300
		Expected Count	152.0	148.0	300.0

Figure IV-75 Distribution of Frequencies of Blisters between Team and Individual Games

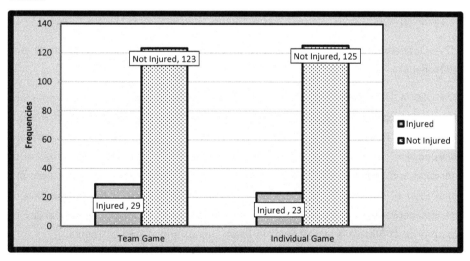

Table IV-81 Comparison between Observed and Expected Frequencies of Blisters

	Chi-Square Tests				
	Value	df	Asymp. Sig. (2-sided)	Exact Sig. (2-sided)	Exact Sig. (1-sided)
Pearson Chi-Square	.655[a]	1	.418		
Continuity Correction[b]	.432	1	.511		
Likelihood Ratio	.657	1	.418		
Fisher's Exact Test				.448	.256
Linear-by-Linear Association	.653	1	.419		
N of Valid Cases	300				

a. 0 cells (0.0%) have expected count less than 5. The minimum expected count is 25.65.

b. Computed only for a 2x2 table

$H2_0$= **Occurrence of Blisters and type of sports are independent** - there is no relationship.

$H2_1$= **Occurrence of Blisters and type of sports are not independent** - there is a relationship.

The table 4.81 revealed that association found between Blisters and Game Type is not strong. The calculated value of χ^2 (.655) is less than the table value (3.84) at P ≥ 0.5 level, df =1. The null hypothesis (H_0) "*Occurrence of Abrasion and type of sports are independent*" thus, is accepted while alternative hypothesis (H_1) "*Occurrence of Abrasion and type of sports are not independent*" is rejected. This is evident from the illustration of table 4.80 that there is no significant difference in the frequencies of Blisters between the team and individual sportspersons. It means the probability of occurrence of Blisters is almost same in Team Games and Individual Games.

Table IV-82 Cross Tabulation of Frequencies of Contusion between Team and Individual Game

			Crosstab		
			GAME TYPE		Total
			Team Game	Individual Game	
Contusion	Not Injured	Count	96	102	198
		Expected Count	100.3	97.7	198.0
	Injured	Count	56	46	102
		Expected Count	51.7	50.3	102.0
Total		Count	152	148	300
		Expected Count	152.0	148.0	300.0

Figure IV-76 Distribution of Frequencies of Contusion between Team and Individual Games

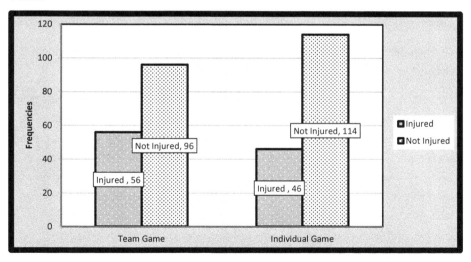

Table IV-83 Comparison between Observed and Expected Frequencies of Contusion

	Chi-Square Tests				
	Value	df	Asymp. Sig. (2-sided)	Exact Sig. (2-sided)	Exact Sig. (1-sided)
Pearson Chi-Square	1.109[a]	1	.292		
Continuity Correction[b]	.867	1	.352		
Likelihood Ratio	1.110	1	.292		
Fisher's Exact Test				.330	.176
Linear-by-Linear Association	1.105	1	.293		
N of Valid Cases	300				

a. 0 cells (0.0%) have expected count less than 5. The minimum expected count is 50.32.

b. Computed only for a 2x2 table

$H3_0$= **Occurrence of Contusion and type of sports are independent** - there is no relationship.

$H3_1$= **Occurrence of Contusion and type of sports are not independent** - there is a relationship.

The table 4.83 revealed that association found between Blisters and Game Type is not strong. The calculated value of χ^2 (1.109) is less than the table value (3.84) at $P \geq 0.5$ level, df =1. The null hypothesis (H_0) "*Occurrence of Contusion and type of sports are independent*" thus, is accepted while alternative hypothesis (H_1) "*Occurrence of Contusion and type of sports are not independent*" is rejected. This is evident from the illustration of table 4.82 that there is no significant difference in the frequencies of Contusion between the team and individual sportspersons. It means the probability of occurrence of Contusion is almost same in Team Games and Individual Games.

Table IV-84 Cross Tabulation of Frequencies of Incision between Team and Individual Game

			GAME TYPE		Total
			Team Game	Individual Game	
Incision	Not Injured	Count	119	134	253
		Expected Count	128.2	124.8	253.0
	Injured	Count	33	14	47
		Expected Count	23.8	23.2	47.0
Total		Count	152	148	300
		Expected Count	152.0	148.0	300.0

Figure IV-77 Distribution of Frequencies of Incision between Team and Individual Games

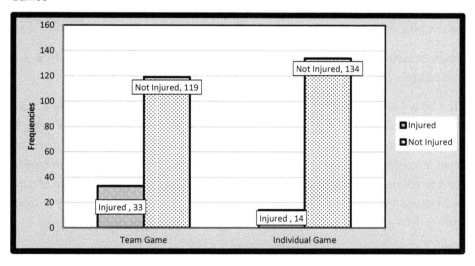

Table IV-85 Comparison between Observed and Expected Frequencies of Incision

	Value	df	Asymp. Sig. (2-sided)	Exact Sig. (2-sided)	Exact Sig. (1-sided)
		Chi-Square Tests			
Pearson Chi-Square	8.518[a]	1	.004		
Continuity Correction[b]	7.616	1	.006		
Likelihood Ratio	8.742	1	.003		
Fisher's Exact Test				.004	.003
Linear-by-Linear Association	8.490	1	.004		
N of Valid Cases	300				

a. 0 cells (0.0%) have expected count less than 5. The minimum expected count is 23.19.

b. Computed only for a 2x2 table

$H4_0$= **Occurrence of Incision and type of sports are independent** - there is no relationship.

$H4_1$= **Occurrence of Incision and type of sports are not independent** - there is a relationship.

The table 4.85 revealed that the association between Incision and Game Type is high. The calculated value of χ^2 (8.518) is more than the table value (3.84) at P ≤ 0.5 level, df =1. The null hypothesis (H_0) "Occurrence of Incision and type of sports are independent" thus, is rejected while alternative hypothesis **(H_1) "Occurrence of Incision and type of sports are not independent"** **is accepted**. This is evident from the illustration of table 4.84 where the highest frequencies of injured respondents are come from the Team games. It means the probability of occurrence of Incision is higher in Team Games.

Table IV-86 Cross Tabulation of Frequencies of Laceration between Team and Individual Game

Crosstab

			GAME TYPE		Total
			Team Game	Individual Game	
Laceration	Not Injured	Count	129	141	270
		Expected Count	136.8	133.2	270.0
	Injured	Count	23	7	30
		Expected Count	15.2	14.8	30.0
Total		Count	152	148	300
		Expected Count	152.0	148.0	300.0

Figure IV-78 Distribution of Frequencies of Laceration between Team and Individual Games

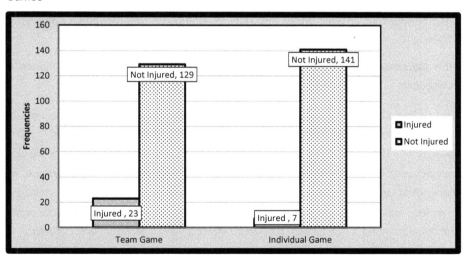

Table IV-87 Comparison between Observed and Expected Frequencies of Laceration

| | **Chi-Square Tests** | | | | |
	Value	**df**	**Asymp. Sig. (2-sided)**	**Exact Sig. (2-sided)**	**Exact Sig. (1-sided)**
Pearson Chi-Square	**9.015[a]**	**1**	**.003**		
Continuity Correction[b]	7.896	1	.005		
Likelihood Ratio	9.473	1	.002		
Fisher's Exact Test				.003	.002
Linear-by-Linear Association	8.985	1	.003		
N of Valid Cases	300				

a. 0 cells (0.0%) have expected count less than 5. The minimum expected count is 14.80.

b. Computed only for a 2x2 table

$H5_0$= **Occurrence of Laceration and type of sports are independent** - there is no relationship.

$H5_1$= **Occurrence of Laceration and type of sports are not independent** - there is a relationship.

The table 4.87 revealed that the association between Laceration and Game Type is high. The calculated value of χ^2 (9.015) is more than the table value (3.84) at $P \leq 0.5$ level, df =1. The null hypothesis (H_0) "Occurrence of Laceration and type of sports are independent" thus, is rejected while alternative hypothesis **(H_1) "Occurrence of Laceration and type of sports are not independent" is accepted.** This is evident from the illustration of table 4.86 where the highest frequencies of injured respondents are come from the Team games. It means the probability of occurrence of Laceration is higher in Team Games.

Table IV-88 Cross Tabulation of Frequencies of Dislocation between Team and Individual Game

Crosstab			GAME TYPE		Total
			Team Game	Individual Game	
Dislocation	Not Injured	Count	135	122	257
		Expected Count	130.2	126.8	257.0
	Injured	Count	17	26	43
		Expected Count	21.8	21.2	43.0
Total		Count	152	148	300
		Expected Count	152.0	148.0	300.0

Figure IV-79 Distribution of Frequencies of Dislocation between Team and Individual Games

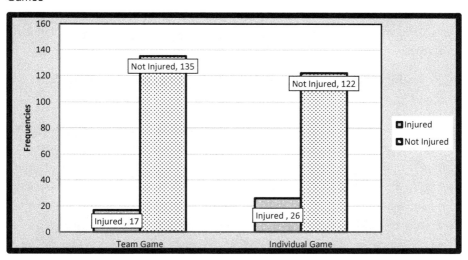

Table IV-89 Comparison between Observed and Expected Frequencies of Dislocation

	Chi-Square Tests				
	Value	df	Asymp. Sig. (2-sided)	Exact Sig. (2-sided)	Exact Sig. (1-sided)
Pearson Chi-Square	**2.488**[a]	**1**	**.115**		
Continuity Correction[b]	1.996	1	.158		
Likelihood Ratio	2.502	1	.114		
Fisher's Exact Test				.138	.079
Linear-by-Linear Association	2.480	1	.115		
N of Valid Cases	300				

a. 0 cells (0.0%) have expected count less than 5. The minimum expected count is 21.21.

b. Computed only for a 2x2 table

H6$_0$= **Occurrence of Dislocation and type of sports are independent** - there is no relationship.

H6$_1$= **Occurrence of Dislocation and type of sports are not independent** - there is a relationship.

The table 4.89 revealed that association found between Blisters and Game Type is not strong. The calculated value of χ^2 (2.448) is less than the table value (3.84) at P ≥ 0.5 level, df =1. The null hypothesis **(H$_0$)** *"Occurrence of Dislocation and type of sports are independent"* **thus, is accepted** while alternative hypothesis (H$_1$) "*Occurrence of Abrasion and type of sports are not independent*" is rejected. This is evident from the illustration of table 4.88 that there is no significant difference in the frequencies of Dislocation between the team and individual sportspersons. It means the probability of occurrence of Dislocation is almost same in Team Games and Individual Games.

Table IV-90 Cross Tabulation of Frequencies of Fracture between Team and Individual Game

Crosstab			GAME TYPE		Total
			Team Game	Individual Game	
Fracture	Not Injured	Count	111	112	223
		Expected Count	113.0	110.0	223.0
	Injured	Count	41	36	77
		Expected Count	39.0	38.0	77.0
Total		Count	152	148	300
		Expected Count	152.0	148.0	300.0

Figure IV-80 Distribution of Frequencies of Fracture between Team and Individual Games

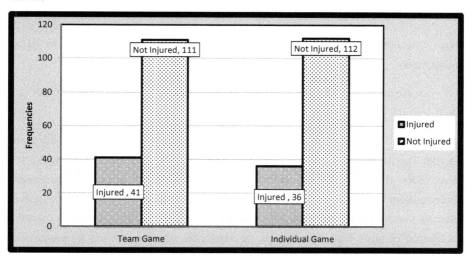

Table IV-91 Comparison between Observed and Expected Frequencies of Fracture

		Chi-Square Tests			
	Value	df	Asymp. Sig. (2-sided)	Exact Sig. (2-sided)	Exact Sig. (1-sided)
Pearson Chi-Square	.276[a]	1	.599		
Continuity Correction[b]	.154	1	.694		
Likelihood Ratio	.276	1	.599		
Fisher's Exact Test				.692	.347
Linear-by-Linear Association	.275	1	.600		
N of Valid Cases	300				

a. 0 cells (0.0%) have expected count less than 5. The minimum expected count is 37.99.

b. Computed only for a 2x2 table

$H7_0$= **Occurrence of Fracture and type of sports are independent** - there is no relationship.

$H7_1$= **Occurrence of Fracture and type of sports are not independent** - there is a relationship.

The table 4.91 revealed that association found between Blisters and Game Type is not strong. The calculated value of χ^2 (0.276) is less than the table value (3.84) at P ≥ 0.5 level, df =1. The null hypothesis **(H_0)** *"Occurrence of Abrasion and type of sports are independent"* **thus, is accepted** while alternative hypothesis (H_1) "*Occurrence of Abrasion and type of sports are not independent*" is rejected. This is evident from the illustration of table 4.90 that there is no significant difference in the frequencies of Fractures between the team and individual sportspersons. It means the probability of occurrence of Fractures is almost same in Team Games and Individual Games.

Table IV-92 Cross Tabulation of Frequencies of Ligament Rupture between Team and Individual Game

Crosstab					
			GAME TYPE		Total
			Team Game	Individual Game	
Ligament Rupture	Not Injured	Count	123	125	248
		Expected Count	125.7	122.3	248.0
	Injured	Count	29	23	52
		Expected Count	26.3	25.7	52.0
Total		Count	152	148	300
		Expected Count	152.0	148.0	300.0

Figure IV-81 Distribution of Frequencies of Ligament Rupture between Team and Individual Games

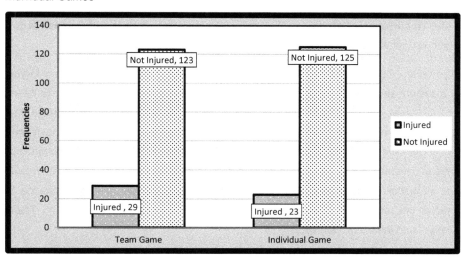

Table IV-93 Comparison between Observed and Expected Frequencies of ligament Rupture

	Chi-Square Tests				
	Value	df	Asymp. Sig. (2-sided)	Exact Sig. (2-sided)	Exact Sig. (1-sided)
Pearson Chi-Square	**.655**[a]	**1**	**.418**		
Continuity Correction[b]	.432	1	.511		
Likelihood Ratio	.657	1	.418		
Fisher's Exact Test				.448	.256
Linear-by-Linear Association	.653	1	.419		
N of Valid Cases	300				

a. 0 cells (0.0%) have expected count less than 5. The minimum expected count is 25.65.

b. Computed only for a 2x2 table

$H8_0$= **Occurrence of Ligament Rupture and type of sports are independent** - there is no relationship.

$H8_1$= **Occurrence of Ligament Rupture and type of sports are not independent** - there is a relationship.

The table 4.93 revealed that association found between Ligament Rupture and Game Type is not strong. The calculated value of χ^2 (.655) is less than the table value (3.84) at $P \geq 0.5$ level, df =1. The null hypothesis **(H_0)** *"Occurrence of Ligament Rupture and type of sports are independent"* **thus, is accepted** while alternative hypothesis (H_1) *"Occurrence of Ligament Rupture and type of sports are not independent"* is rejected. This is evident from the illustration of table 4.92 that there is no significant difference in the frequencies of Ligament Rupture between the team and individual sportspersons. It means the probability of occurrence of Ligament Rupture is almost same in Team Games and Individual Games.

Table IV-94 Cross Tabulation of Frequencies of Muscle Cramp between Team and Individual Game

Crosstab					
			GAME TYPE		Total
			Team Game	Individual Game	
Muscle Cramp	Not Injured	Count	118	115	233
		Expected Count	118.1	114.9	233.0
	Injured	Count	34	33	67
		Expected Count	33.9	33.1	67.0
Total		Count	152	148	300
		Expected Count	152.0	148.0	300.0

Figure IV-82 Distribution of Frequencies of Muscle Cramp between Team and Individual Games

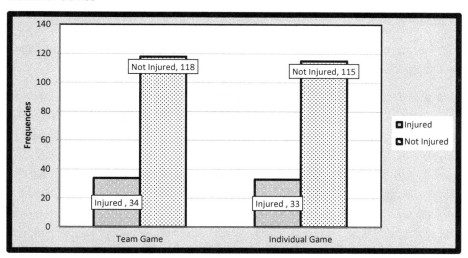

Table IV-95 Comparison between Observed and Expected Frequencies of Muscle Cramp

	Chi-Square Tests				
	Value	df	Asymp. Sig. (2-sided)	Exact Sig. (2-sided)	Exact Sig. (1-sided)
Pearson Chi-Square	.000[a]	1	.988		
Continuity Correction[b]	.000	1	1.000		
Likelihood Ratio	.000	1	.988		
Fisher's Exact Test				1.000	.549
Linear-by-Linear Association	.000	1	.988		
N of Valid Cases	300				

a. 0 cells (0.0%) have expected count less than 5. The minimum expected count is 33.05.

b. Computed only for a 2x2 table

H9$_0$= **Occurrence of Muscle Cramp and type of sports are independent** - there is no relationship.

H9$_1$= **Occurrence of Muscle Cramp and type of sports are not independent** - there is a relationship.

The table 4.95 revealed that association found between Muscle Cramp and Game Type is not strong. The calculated value of χ^2 (.000) is less than the table value (3.84) at P ≥ 0.5 level, df =1. The null hypothesis **(H$_0$)** *"Occurrence of Muscle Cramp and type of sports are independent"* **thus, is accepted** while alternative hypothesis (H$_1$) *"Occurrence of Muscle Cramp and type of sports are not independent"* is rejected. This is evident from the illustration of table 4.94 that there is no significant difference in the frequencies of Muscle Cramp between the team and individual sportspersons. It means the probability of occurrence of Muscle Cramp is almost same in Team Games and Individual Games.

Table IV-96 Cross Tabulation of Frequencies of Muscle Pull between Team and Individual Game

Crosstab					
			GAME TYPE		Total
			Team Game	Individual Game	
Muscle Pull	Not Injured	Count	95	97	192
		Expected Count	97.3	94.7	192.0
	Injured	Count	57	51	108
		Expected Count	54.7	53.3	108.0
Total		Count	152	148	300
		Expected Count	152.0	148.0	300.0

Figure IV-83 Distribution of Frequencies of Muscle Pull between Team and Individual Games

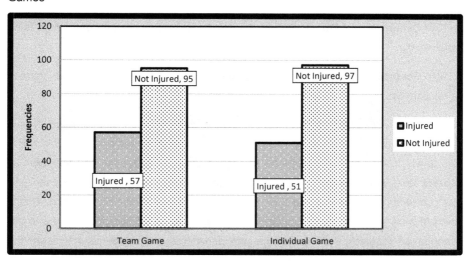

Table IV-97 Comparison between Observed and Expected Frequencies of Muscle Pull

	Chi-Square Tests				
	Value	**df**	**Asymp. Sig. (2-sided)**	**Exact Sig. (2-sided)**	**Exact Sig. (1-sided)**
Pearson Chi-Square	.301[a]	1	.583		
Continuity Correction[b]	.183	1	.668		
Likelihood Ratio	.301	1	.583		
Fisher's Exact Test				.631	.334
Linear-by-Linear Association	.300	1	.584		
N of Valid Cases	300				

a. 0 cells (0.0%) have expected count less than 5. The minimum expected count is 53.28.

b. Computed only for a 2x2 table

H10$_0$= **Occurrence of Muscle Pull and type of sports are independent** - there is no relationship.

H10$_1$= **Occurrence of Muscle Pull and type of sports are not independent** - there is a relationship.

The table 4.97 revealed that association found between Muscle Pull and Game Type is not strong. The calculated value of χ^2 (.0.301) is less than the table value (3.84) at P ≥ 0.5 level, df =1. The null hypothesis **(H$_0$) "Occurrence of Muscle Pull and type of sports are independent" thus, is accepted** while alternative hypothesis (H$_1$) "Occurrence of Muscle Pull and type of sports are not independent" is rejected. This is evident from the illustration of table 4.96 that there is no significant difference in the frequencies of Muscle Pull between the team and individual sportspersons. It means the probability of occurrence of Muscle Pull is almost same in Team Games and Individual Games.

Table IV-98 Cross Tabulation of Frequencies of Puncture Wound between Team and Individual Game

Crosstab			GAME TYPE		Total
			Team Game	Individual Game	
Puncture Wound	Not Injured	Count	149	148	297
		Expected Count	150.5	146.5	297.0
	Injured	Count	3	0	3
		Expected Count	1.5	1.5	3.0
Total		Count	152	148	300
		Expected Count	152.0	148.0	300.0

Figure IV-84 Distribution of Frequencies of Puncture Wound between Team and Individual Games

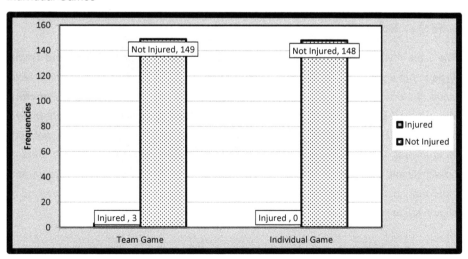

Table IV-99 Comparison between Observed and Expected Frequencies of Puncture Wound

	Chi-Square Tests				
	Value	df	Asymp. Sig. (2-sided)	Exact Sig. (2-sided)	Exact Sig. (1-sided)
Pearson Chi-Square	**2.951**[a]	**1**	**.086**		
Continuity Correction[b]	1.294	1	.255		
Likelihood Ratio	4.109	1	.043		
Fisher's Exact Test				.248	.129
Linear-by-Linear Association	2.941	1	.086		
N of Valid Cases	300				

a. 2 cells (50.0%) have expected count less than 5. The minimum expected count is 1.48.

b. Computed only for a 2x2 table

H11$_0$= **Occurrence of Puncture Wound and type of sports are independent** - there is no relationship.

H11$_1$= **Occurrence of Puncture Wound and type of sports are not independent** - there is a relationship.

The table 4.99 revealed that association found between Puncture Wound and Game Type is not statistically strong. The calculated value of χ^2 (2.951) is less than the table value (3.84) at P ≥ 0.5 level, df =1. The null hypothesis **(H$_0$) "Occurrence of Puncture Wound and type of sports are independent"** thus, **is accepted** while alternative hypothesis (H$_1$) "Occurrence of Puncture Wound and type of sports are not independent" is rejected. This is evident from the illustration of table 4.98 that there is no significant difference in the frequencies of Puncture Wound between the team and individual sportspersons. It means the probability of occurrence of Puncture Wound is almost same in Team Games and Individual Games.

Table IV-100 Cross Tabulation of Frequencies of Sprain between Team and Individual Game

			GAME TYPE		Total
		Crosstab	Team Game	Individual Game	
Sprain	Not Injured	Count	85	112	197
		Expected Count	99.8	97.2	197.0
	Injured	Count	67	36	103
		Expected Count	52.2	50.8	103.0
Total		Count	152	148	300
		Expected Count	152.0	148.0	300.0

Figure IV-85 Distribution of Frequencies of Sprain between Team and Individual Games

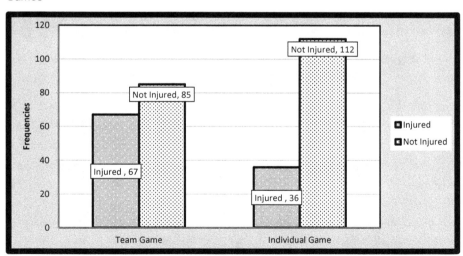

Table IV-101 Comparison between Observed and Expected Frequencies of Sprain

	Chi-Square Tests				
	Value	df	Asymp. Sig. (2-sided)	Exact Sig. (2-sided)	Exact Sig. (1-sided)
Pearson Chi-Square	12.980[a]	1	.000		
Continuity Correction[b]	12.118	1	.000		
Likelihood Ratio	13.135	1	.000		
Fisher's Exact Test				.000	.000
Linear-by-Linear Association	12.936	1	.000		
N of Valid Cases	300				

a. 0 cells (0.0%) have expected count less than 5. The minimum expected count is 50.81.

b. Computed only for a 2x2 table

$H12_0$= **Occurrence of Sprain and type of sports are independent** - there is no relationship.

$H12_1$= **Occurrence of Sprain and type of sports are not independent** - there is a relationship.

The table 4.101 revealed that the association between Sprain and Game Type is high. The calculated value of χ^2 (12.980) is more than the table value (3.84) at $P \leq 0.5$ level, df =1. The null hypothesis (H_0) "Occurrence of Sprain and type of sports are independent" thus, is rejected while alternative hypothesis **(H_1)** *"Occurrence of Sprain and type of sports are not independent"* **is accepted.** This is evident from the illustration of table 4.100 where the highest frequencies of injured respondents are come from the Team games. It means the probability of occurrence of Sprain is higher in Team Games.

Table IV-102 Cross Tabulation of Frequencies of Strain between Team and Individual Game

			GAME TYPE		Total
		Crosstab	**Team Game**	**Individual Game**	**Total**
Strain	Not Injured	Count	115	126	241
		Expected Count	122.1	118.9	241.0
	Injured	Count	37	22	59
		Expected Count	29.9	29.1	59.0
Total		Count	152	148	300
		Expected Count	152.0	148.0	300.0

Figure IV-86 Distribution of Frequencies of Stain between Team and Individual Games

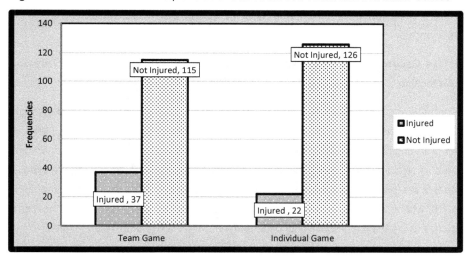

Table IV-103 Comparison between Observed and Expected Frequencies of Strain

	Chi-Square Tests				
	Value	df	Asymp. Sig. (2-sided)	Exact Sig. (2-sided)	Exact Sig. (1-sided)
Pearson Chi-Square	4.263[a]	1	.039		
Continuity Correction[b]	3.684	1	.055		
Likelihood Ratio	4.305	1	.038		
Fisher's Exact Test				.043	.027
Linear-by-Linear Association	4.249	1	.039		
N of Valid Cases	300				

a. 0 cells (0.0%) have expected count less than 5. The minimum expected count is 29.11.

b. Computed only for a 2x2 table

H13$_0$= **Occurrence of Strain and type of sports are independent** - there is no relationship.

H13$_1$= **Occurrence of Strain and type of sports are not independent** - there is a relationship.

The table 4.103 revealed that the association between Strain and Game Type is high. The calculated value of χ^2 (4.263) is more than the table value (3.84) at P ≤ 0.5 level, df =1. The null hypothesis (H$_0$) "Occurrence of Strain and type of sports are independent" thus, is rejected while alternative hypothesis **(H$_1$)** *"Occurrence of Strain and type of sports are not independent"* **is accepted.** This is evident from the illustration of table 4.102 where the highest frequencies of injured respondents are come from the Team games. It means the probability of occurrence of Strain is higher in Team Games.

Table IV-104 Cross Tabulation of Frequencies of Tendinitis between Team and Individual Game

		Crosstab			
			GAME TYPE		Total
			Team Game	Individual Game	
Tendinitis	Not Injured	Count	147	147	294
		Expected Count	149.0	145.0	294.0
	Injured	Count	5	1	6
		Expected Count	3.0	3.0	6.0
Total		Count	152	148	300
		Expected Count	152.0	148.0	300.0

Figure IV-87 Distribution of Frequencies of Tendinitis between Team and Individual Games

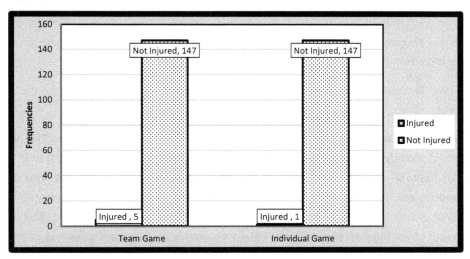

Table IV-105 Comparison between Observed and Expected Frequencies of Tendinitis

	Value	df	Chi-Square Tests Asymp. Sig. (2-sided)	Exact Sig. (2-sided)	Exact Sig. (1-sided)
Pearson Chi-Square	2.614^a	1	.106		
Continuity Correction[b]	1.450	1	.228		
Likelihood Ratio	2.858	1	.091		
Fisher's Exact Test				.214	.113
Linear-by-Linear Association	2.605	1	.107		
N of Valid Cases	300				

a. 2 cells (50.0%) have expected count less than 5. The minimum expected count is 2.96.

b. Computed only for a 2x2 table

$H14_0$= **Occurrence of Tendonitis and type of sports are independent** - there is no relationship.

$H14_1$= **Occurrence of Tendonitis and type of sports are not independent** - there is a relationship.

The table 4.105 revealed that association found between Tendonitis and Game Type is not strong. The calculated value of χ^2 (2.614) is less than the table value (3.84) at $P \geq$ 0.5 level, df =1. The null hypothesis **(H_0) "Occurrence of Tendonitis and type of sports are independent" thus, is accepted** while alternative hypothesis (H_1) "Occurrence of Tendonitis and type of sports are not independent" is rejected. This is evident from the illustration of table 4.104 that there is no significant difference in the frequencies of Tendonitis between the team and individual sportspersons. It means the probability of occurrence of Tendonitis is almost same in Team Games and Individual Games.

Table IV-106 Cross Tabulation of Frequencies of Concussion between Team and Individual Game

			GAME TYPE		Total
Crosstab					
			Team Game	**Individual Game**	**Total**
Concussion	Not Injured	Count	148	148	296
		Expected Count	150.0	146.0	296.0
	Injured	Count	4	0	4
		Expected Count	2.0	2.0	4.0
Total		Count	152	148	300
		Expected Count	152.0	148.0	300.0

Figure IV-88 Distribution of Frequencies of Concussion between Team and Individual Games

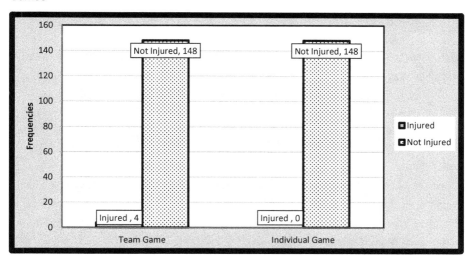

Table IV-107 Comparison between Observed and Expected Frequencies of Concussion

	Chi-Square Tests				
	Value	df	Asymp. Sig. (2-sided)	Exact Sig. (2-sided)	Exact Sig. (1-sided)
Pearson Chi-Square	3.947[a]	1	.047		
Continuity Correction[b]	2.200	1	.138		
Likelihood Ratio	5.492	1	.019		
Fisher's Exact Test				.123	.065
Linear-by-Linear Association	3.934	1	.047		
N of Valid Cases	300				

a. 2 cells (50.0%) have expected count less than 5. The minimum expected count is 1.97.

b. Computed only for a 2x2 table

$H15_0$= **Occurrence of Concussion and type of sports are independent** - there is no relationship.

$H15_1$= **Occurrence of Concussion and type of sports are not independent** - there is a relationship.

The table 4.107 revealed that the association between Concussion and Game Type is high. The calculated value of χ^2 (3.947) is more than the table value (3.84) at $P \leq 0.5$ level, df =1. The null hypothesis (H_0) "Occurrence of Concussion and type of sports are independent" thus, is rejected while alternative hypothesis **(H_1) "Occurrence of Concussion and type of sports are not independent"** is accepted. This is evident from the illustration of table 4.106 where the highest frequencies of injured respondents are come from the Team games. It means the probability of occurrence of Concussion is higher in Team Games.

Table IV-108 Cross Tabulation of Frequencies of Meniscus Tear between Team and Individual Game

Crosstab			GAME TYPE		Total
			Team Game	Individual Game	
Meniscus Tear	Not Injured	Count	146	146	292
		Expected Count	147.9	144.1	292.0
	Injured	Count	6	2	8
		Expected Count	4.1	3.9	8.0
Total		Count	152	148	300
		Expected Count	152.0	148.0	300.0

Figure IV-89 Distribution of Frequencies of Meniscus Tear between Team and Individual Games

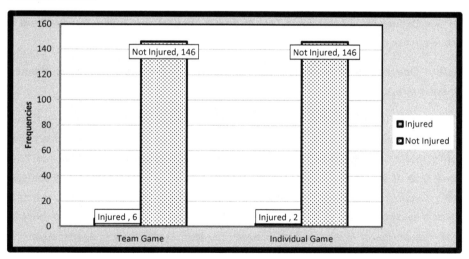

Table IV-109 Comparison between Observed and Expected Frequencies of Meniscus Tear

	Chi-Square Tests				
	Value	df	Asymp. Sig. (2-sided)	Exact Sig. (2-sided)	Exact Sig. (1-sided)
Pearson Chi-Square	1.947[a]	1	.163		
Continuity Correction[b]	1.075	1	.300		
Likelihood Ratio	2.040	1	.153		
Fisher's Exact Test				.283	.150
Linear-by-Linear Association	1.941	1	.164		
N of Valid Cases	300				

a. 2 cells (50.0%) have expected count less than 5. The minimum expected count is 3.95.

b. Computed only for a 2x2 table

$H16_0$= **Occurrence of Meniscus Tear and type of sports are independent** - there is no relationship.

$H16_1$= **Occurrence of Meniscus Tear and type of sports are not independent** - there is a relationship.

The table 4.109 revealed that association found between Meniscus Tear and Game Type is not strong. The calculated value of χ^2 (1.947) is less than the table value (3.84) at P(.163) $\geq$ 0.5 level, df =1. The null hypothesis **(H_0) "Occurrence of Meniscus Tear and type of sports are independent" thus, is accepted** while alternative hypothesis (H_1) "Occurrence of Meniscus Tear and type of sports are not independent" is rejected. This is evident from the illustration of table 4.108 that there is no significant difference in the frequencies of Meniscus Tear between the team and individual sportspersons. It means the probability of occurrence of Meniscus Tear is almost same in Team Games and Individual Games.

Table IV-110 Cross Tabulation of Frequencies of Back Pain between Team and Individual Game

		Crosstab			
			GAME TYPE		Total
			Team Game	Individual Game	
BACK PAIN	Not Injured	Count	149	142	291
		Expected Count	147.4	143.6	291.0
	Injured	Count	3	6	9
		Expected Count	4.6	4.4	9.0
Total		Count	152	148	300
		Expected Count	152.0	148.0	300.0

Figure IV-90 Distribution of Frequencies of Back Pain between Team and Individual Games

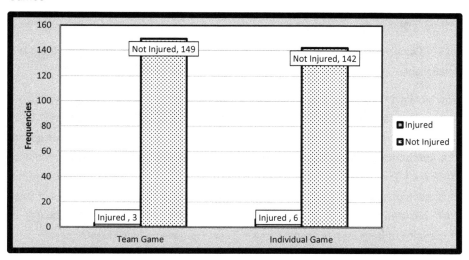

Table IV-111 Comparison between Observed and Expected Frequencies of Back Pain

	Chi-Square Tests				
	Value	df	Asymp. Sig. (2-sided)	Exact Sig. (2-sided)	Exact Sig. (1-sided)
Pearson Chi-Square	1.115[a]	1	.291		
Continuity Correction[b]	.515	1	.473		
Likelihood Ratio	1.134	1	.287		
Fisher's Exact Test				.331	.238
Linear-by-Linear Association	1.112	1	.292		
N of Valid Cases	300				

a. 2 cells (50.0%) have expected count less than 5. The minimum expected count is 4.44.

b. Computed only for a 2x2 table

$H17_0$= **Occurrence of Back Pain and type of sports are independent** - there is no relationship.

$H17_1$= **Occurrence of Back Pain and type of sports are not independent** - there is a relationship.

The table 4.111 revealed that association found between Blisters and Game Type is not strong. The calculated value of χ^2 (1.115) is less than the table value (3.84) at $P \geq 0.5$ level, df =1. The null hypothesis **(H_0) "*Occurrence of* Back Pain *and type of sports are independent*" thus, is accepted** while alternative hypothesis (H_1) "*Occurrence of Back Pain and type of sports are not independent*" is rejected. This is evident from the illustration of table 4.110 that there is no significant difference in the frequencies of Back Pain between the team and individual sportspersons. It means the probability of occurrence of Back Pain is almost same in Team Games and Individual Games.

Table IV-112 Cross Tabulation of Frequencies of Muscle Tear between Team and Individual Game

Crosstab			GAME TYPE		Total
			Team Game	Individual Game	
MUSCLE TEAR	Not Injured	Count	150	148	298
		Expected Count	151.0	147.0	298.0
	Injured	Count	2	0	2
		Expected Count	1.0	1.0	2.0
Total		Count	152	148	300
		Expected Count	152.0	148.0	300.0

Figure IV-91 Distribution of Frequencies of Muscle Tear between Team and Individual Games

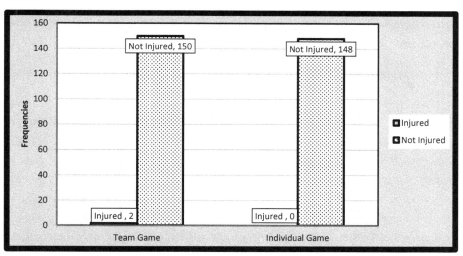

Table IV-113 Comparison between Observed and Expected Frequencies of Muscle Tear

| | Chi-Square Tests | | | | |
	Value	df	Asymp. Sig. (2-sided)	Exact Sig. (2-sided)	Exact Sig. (1-sided)
Pearson Chi-Square	1.960[a]	1	.161		
Continuity Correction[b]	.477	1	.490		
Likelihood Ratio	2.733	1	.098		
Fisher's Exact Test				.498	.256
Linear-by-Linear Association	1.954	1	.162		
N of Valid Cases	300				

a. 2 cells (50.0%) have expected count less than 5. The minimum expected count is .99.

b. Computed only for a 2x2 table

$H18_0$= **Occurrence of Muscle Tear and type of sports are independent** - there is no relationship.

$H18_1$= **Occurrence of Muscle Tear and type of sports are not independent** - there is a relationship.

The table 4.113 revealed that association found between Muscle Tear and Game Type is not strong. The calculated value of χ^2 (1.960) is less than the table value (3.84) at P ≥ 0.5 level, df =1. The null hypothesis **(H₀)** *"Occurrence of **Muscle Tear** **and type of sports are independent"** thus, is accepted* while alternative hypothesis (H₁) *"Occurrence of Muscle Tear and type of sports are not independent"* is rejected. This is evident from the illustration of table 4.112 that there is no significant difference in the frequencies of Muscle Tear between the team and individual sportspersons. It means the probability of occurrence of Muscle Tear is almost same in Team Games and Individual Games.

Table IV-114 Cross Tabulation of Frequencies of Rotator Cuff between Team and Individual Game

		Crosstab			
			GAME TYPE		**Total**
			Team Game	**Individual Game**	
Rotator Cuff	Not Injured	Count	145	145	290
		Expected Count	146.9	143.1	290.0
	Injured	Count	7	3	10
		Expected Count	5.1	4.9	10.0
Total		Count	152	148	300
		Expected Count	152.0	148.0	300.0

Figure IV-92 Distribution of Frequencies of Rotator Cuff between Team and Individual Games

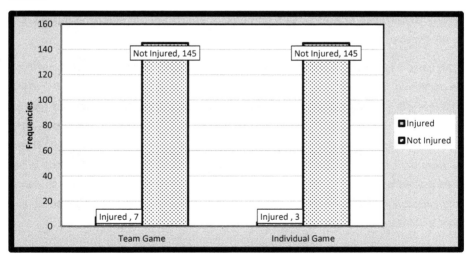

220

Table IV-115 Comparison between Observed and Expected Frequencies of Rotator Cuff

| | **Chi-Square Tests** | | | | |
	Value	**df**	**Asymp. Sig. (2-sided)**	**Exact Sig. (2-sided)**	**Exact Sig. (1-sided)**
Pearson Chi-Square	1.547[a]	1	.214		
Continuity Correction[b]	.850	1	.356		
Likelihood Ratio	1.592	1	.207		
Fisher's Exact Test				.336	.179
Linear-by-Linear Association	1.542	1	.214		
N of Valid Cases	300				

a. 1 cells (25.0%) have expected count less than 5. The minimum expected count is 4.93.

b. Computed only for a 2x2 table

$H19_0=$ **Occurrence of Rotator Cuff and type of sports are independent** - there is no relationship.

$H19_1=$ **Occurrence of Rotator Cuff and type of sports are not independent** - there is a relationship.

The table 4.115 revealed that association found between Rotator Cuff and Game Type is not strong. The calculated value of χ^2 (1.547) is less than the table value (3.84) at P ≥ 0.5 level, df =1. The null hypothesis (H_0) **"Occurrence of Rotator Cuff and type of sports are independent" thus, is accepted** while alternative hypothesis (H_1) "Occurrence of Rotator Cuff and type of sports are not independent" is rejected. This is evident from the illustration of table 4.114 that there is no significant difference in the frequencies of Rotator Cuff between the team and individual sportspersons. It means the probability of occurrence of Rotator Cuff is almost same in Team Games and Individual Games.

Chapter-V

SUMMARY, CONCLUSION AND RECOMMENDATION

Chapter-V

SUMMARY, CONCLUSIONS AND RECOMMENDATIONS

Overview

Chapter-V

SUMMARY, CONCLUSIONS AND RECOMMENDATIONS

V. Summary, Conclusion and Recommendation

V.1 SUMMARY

This study made a systematic attempt focusing on common sports injuries between Team and Individual male sportspersons. In India, the field of sports injury or sports medicine is a challengeable task for a researcher. In India, sports lack valid injury data collection framework. On the school or college level there is no space for sports medicine as a subject in our curriculum. So, the area of injury prevention and management is unidentified, neglected and unrecognized one. There is not a single register in stadium or sports clubs to record the history of sports injuries of participants. During data collection it was observed that mostly of the sportsperson did not know the meaning of 'Sprain' as well. Researcher personally visit some reputed sports injury centers to collect reliable and secondary data but they did not have enough record of sports injuries to do research work. The severity of injury in sports can developed physical and psychological disorder in young individuals whom have a dream to be an elite sportsperson. Occurrences of severe injuries are rarely possible in sports, but neglected severe injury may lead to serious effect on body or death also. So the research on prevention and management of sports injuries and techniques of rehabilitation should be promoted to avoid social disturbance, Economic cost of injury treatment and for the promotion of safe play.

The investigation in this study will bring awareness towards injury prevention and management among coaches, players, organizers, teachers and coaches to recognize which injury relate to which sports and which body parts is highly probable to what type of injury. This examination will add to the current assemblage of information about the investment and gives point by point data about the injuries that a player can sustain in particular sports. The purpose of sports for every participant should be to exploit the activity whether it should be physically, mentally or psychologically and also avoid serious muscoskeletal injuries which may lead serious lifelong consequences. So the researches should have correspondingly pointed to the need for the evaluation of the injury risks and benefits associated with various types of sporting activities.

V.2 FINDINGS

V.2.1 Findings in Distribution of Injuries in Team and Individual Games

Team Games: A total 532 frequencies of injuries were recorded during data collection in team games. Highest, (83) responses are of Abrasion which constitute 15.6% of the total responses. Injury rate (IR) of 'Abrasion' in Team games was 55.7% per 100 athletes. It means if there were 100 injuries occurred in team games then 56 (approximately) should be Abrasion. Second highest, (67) responses are of 'Sprain' which constitute 12.6% of the total responses and Injury rate was 45% respectively. Contusion, Muscle pull, Fracture and Ligament Rupture has also a considerable frequencies and their injury rate illustrate probability of their occurrence. Fracture and Ligament Rupture are severe injuries which may lead serious consequences in the career of a sportsperson. Some Meniscus Tear (1.1%) and Concussion (0.8%) were also observed which are also under the severe category.

Individual Games: A total 364 responses were retraced in Individual Games. Highest, 50 responses were Muscle Pull which constitutes 13.7% of the total responses. Injury rate of muscle pull was 34%, which shows a considerable amount of probability of occurrence in individual games. Second, highest (45) responses were contusion which constitute12.4% of the total sample and out of 100 injuries, the probability of Contusion is 31 approximately. 25 responses were Dislocation which shows a significant amount of injured respondents whose body parts were dislocated in individual games.

Game Wise: Muscle Pull and Abrasions found the highest probable injury in Cricket and Baseball. Sprain is one of the highest frequent injuries in Kabaddi, whereas Fracture and Sprain is frequent injuries in Basketball. Abrasion and Contusion in Hockey, Abrasion, Sprain and Contusion in Football, Fracture and Contusion and Wrestling, Strain and Blisters in Weight Lifting, Muscle Cramp, Muscle Pull and Sprain in Badminton, direct hit on Knuckles (Contusion) in Boxing, Fracture and Abrasion in

Gymnastic, Dislocation and Abrasion in Judo is highest frequent injuries retraced during data collection.

V.2.2 Findings in Body Parts Associated with Injuries

Team Games: Knee is highest frequent body part associated with injuries in team games. A total 415 frequencies of body parts recorded during data collection. 56 responses are Knee which constitutes 13.5% of the total sample and probability of injury occurrence in knee is 48.3% respectively. Second highest responses are come from Ankle. 52 responses are Ankle which constitutes 12.5% of the total responses and probability is 44.8%. Whereas, Elbow, Shoulder, Thigh, Calf, Eyebrow, Hamstring Muscle, Hand, Fingers has also considerable amount of responses noticed.

Individual Games: Knee is found highest body parts associated with injuries Individual Game also. A total 438 responses were noticed. 56 responses are Knee which constitutes 12.8% of the total sample, second, highest body part is Shoulder. 38 responses are Shoulder and which covers 8.7% of the total responses and probability of injury occurrence of shoulder is 27.5% out of hundred times. It is observed that Lumber Vertebrae which is a vital body part has 32 responses which make 7.3% of the total response and probability is 23.2% is a significant amount. Elbow, Fingers, Thigh, Palm, Face, Hamstring Muscle, Wrist, Thumb, Calf, Shin are also found significant association with injuries.

Game Wise: In Cricket Elbow, Lumber Vertebrae and Shoulder have the highest association with injuries. Shoulder is also associated in Baseball also. Knee, elbow, chin and ankle are highly probable to injury in Kabaddi. Ankle and Knee in Basketball, Knee, elbow and hamstring muscle in Hockey, Knee, ankle, thigh, calf, foot in Football, Knee in Wrestling, Lumber Vertebrae in Weight Lifting, Knee, ankle and shoulder in Badminton. Knuckles, nose, thumb and shoulder in Boxing. Shoulder and hand in Gymnastic. Knee, face, ankle and shoulder in Judo found to be most probable body parts associated with injuries. It is observed that mostly responses are come from knee in both team and individual games. It means knee has the highest probability to be injured in both type of games.

V.2.3 Findings in Injury Severity

In previous tables we interpreted only frequency of injury occurrence and most frequent body part associated with injuries. This section brings some important aspect of the present study. There are a huge difference between frequency of injury and severity of an injury. For instance, Abrasion is highest frequent injury in Team and Individual Games but as per the table it has last no. in the table. Severity shows the seriousness of the injury and it was based on the total days lost from practice and competition. It was assumed that an injured person would rest according to their injury severity. More rest mean more serious injury. It was observed that Meniscus Tear is a highest severe injury in Team Games with mean of 150 days lost from competition and practice. Second highest severe is Ligament Rupture within the mean of 129 days approximately. Whereas, the minimum and maximum values of resting days of Ligament rupture are 15±365 days which include partial tear to complete rupture. Next severe injury is fracture. The mean score of fracture is 63.61 days and minimum and maximum rest is 4±180 days which include stress to complicated fractures. Concussion and Low Back Pain are also found significant injuries in team games. In individual Games: Meniscus Tear is also considered severe injury in individual games. But there is a slightly difference in there score of the mean score of meniscus in individual games is 227.50 days (228 approximately). Some meniscus injuries were operated by doctors but after one year of rest and rehabilitation period the pain start again in knee. Mostly of cases told that operation of meniscus tear was not successful. Mean of Dislocation is 83 days in individual games and 34.53 days in team games because in team some subluxate (partial dislocate) were observed but due to the nature of the game complete dislocation were observed in Individual games. The mean score of Fracture is 78.43 which is also higher than the Fracture in Team games. For deep interpretation see table 4-42 in Chatper-4.

After analysis the results it was retraced that frequency of injuries is high in team games but severity of injuries are higher in individual games. Severity are classified on five rating scale on the basis of days lost from competition and practice. With the help of normal curve the score of Injury severity is distributed on three point rating scale (Minor, Moderate, and Severe,) to classified injury severity scale.

225

Figure V-1 Normal Curve Drawn to Develop Three Point Scale for Injury Severity

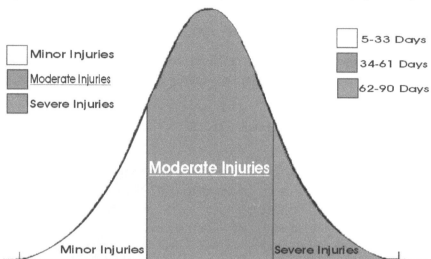

Table V-1 Result for Injury Severity

Days	Severity
5-33	Minor Injuries
34-61	Moderate Injuries
62-90	Severe Injuries

The table 5.1 evident the grading of injury severity on five point rating scale. After injury occurred, if an injured individual will rest 5 to 33 days, his injury will be considered as minor injury. If he rest for 62 to 90 days, his injury will be considered as critical injury.

V.2.4 Findings in Match or Training Injuries

In **team games** a total 458 injuries were recorded. 260 injuries were occurred during match or competition which makes 56.76% of the total responses, whereas 198 injuries were occurred during training period which covered 43.24% of the total response. In **individual games** a total 262 injuries were noticed. 87 injuries were from match which constitute 33.20% of the total responses and 175 injuries were recorded from training which constitute 66.79% of the total sample. So, we can say that in team games the probability of injury occurrence is higher during match in comparison of training on the other hand occurrence of injuries is higher during training in Individual games.

As per **game wise** distribution of injuries, it was observed that Football has the higher rate of injury percentage in both match and training in team games. In individual sports Judo has higher injury prone sports.

V.2.5 Findings in New and Recurrent Injuries

A 'New injury' is defined as an injury which occur first time and 'Recurrent Injury' means, when same injury happens again. The percentage (51.01) of recurrent injuries is higher in team games and percentage distribution of new injuries is higher in individual games. Higher percentage of recurrent injuries shows the injury pattern of team games which show that a same injury is repeating again and again. It could be due to careless and other factors which should be considered in team games. Football and Judo from team and individual games has higher percentage of new and recurrent injuries also.

V.2.6 Findings in Soft Tissue, Bone and Joint Injuries

Football has higher rate of percentage of soft tissue and Joint injuries whereas, Basketball has the highest percentage of bone injuries in team games. In individual games 61 responses of soft tissue injuries were came from Judo which constitutes highest 35.46% of the total responses. 41 responses of frequencies of bone injuries were came from Boxing which covers highest 57.74% of the total responses. In Joint injuries Judo has also highest frequencies (22) which make 36.66% of the total responses. It is recommended that mostly of the injuries could be prevented if an individual use protective equipment's.

V.2.7 Findings in Surface Related Injuries

It was observed that in **team games** clay and natural grass field are highly prone to injuries. A significant amount of injuries were occurred on both surfaces. It was analyzed that wooden surface has the lowest amount of injuries percentage. So, it could be said that playing surface plays a significant role in injury prevention. In individual game highest injury prone surface was Mat. 107 responses of injuries were came from Mat which makes 59.77% of the total responses.

V.2.8 Findings in Injury Reasons

Intrinsic Reason: The reason of injuries was different in various team and individual sports. Improper warming-up is a cause of injury that occurred highest and common in all the sports. Different cause of Injuries in sports varying from one sports to another and affected by various factors. Twisting is a reason of injury that was highest in individual games. It was also an interesting fact that majority of the sportsperson did not know the exact reason of injury that's why they select an option 'Unknown' given in injury report form.

Extrinsic Reason: The various extrinsic reasons were observed in different team and individual sports. Field/playground is a reason of injury that occurred highest in **team games**. This is a very important and considerable reason which can be prevented. At college level sports we have not sufficient and latest facilities for instance, wooden surfaces, artificial grass, AstroTurf etc. The lack of these facilities may lead to injuries in sports. Fall or slip is a second reason that is highest in team games. Careless as a injury reason has also observed considerable responses. It is the part of sports person. When an individual is careless during practice or match then coach duty is to identify the exact reason of their carelessness. In **individual games** collision/impact is a reason of injury that is highest percentage distribution. Second highest extrinsic reason of injury is fall or slip which can be occurred due to various causes such as balance, proper footwear, proper technique, collision etc. it is also observed in extrinsic reasons that some sportsperson did not know the exact reason of injury. That's why a considerable amount of recurrent injuries were noticed in team and individual sports. The knowledge of sports medicine and injury pattern should be essential part of the training of a sports person.

V.2.9 Findings in comparison of sports injuries.

To compare the ordinal data of sports injuries between team and individual sports non-parametric statistics (chi-square) was used.

Table V-2 Association between Injuries and Game Type

Sr.No.	(Injuries)	(df)	(χ^2)	Asymp.sig.
1	Abrasion	1	31.539	.000
2	Blisters	1	.655	.418
3	Contusion	1	1.109	.292
4	Incision	1	8.518	.004
5	Laceration	1	9.015	.003
6	Dislocation	1	2.448	.115
7	Fracture	1	.276	.599
8	Ligament Rupture	1	.655	.418
9	Muscle Cramp	1	.000	.988
10	Muscle Pull	1	.301	.583
11	Puncture wound	1	2.951	.086
12	Sprain	1	12.980	.000
13	Strain	1	4.263	.039
14	Tendonitis	1	2.614	.106
15	Concussion	1	3.947	.047
16	Meniscus tear	1	1.947	.163
17	Low Back Pain	1	1.115	.291
18	Muscle Tear	1	1.960	.161
19	Rotator cuff	1	1.547	.214

The table 5-2 shows the association between injuries and game type. It was observed that association between Abrasion, Incision, Laceration, Sprain, Strain and Concussion and game type is high the value of χ^2 is higher than the table value. It shows that occurrence of these injuries and game types are not independent. In simple words we can says that these significant injuries have the higher probability of occurrence in team games in comparison of individual games.

V.3 CONCLUSIONS

After analysis the whole study following conclusion would be drawn:

- Abrasion and Sprain are more frequent and common injuries in team games.
- Muscle pull, contusion, sprain and fracture are most frequent injuries in individual games.
- Knee, ankle, and shoulder are most frequent and common body part which associated with injuries. Majority of injuries associated with the lower extremities in both the games. The leg is important in weight bearing part for speed in sport, subsequently the knee, ankle joints, foot, the muscles of the upper and lower legs are subjected to the greatest physical pressures that led to injury.
- The finger and wrist are easily injured in activities involving catching and holding of equipment in the events such as Kabaddi, Basket Ball, Badminton and in Hockey due to hit to fingers through a bouncing Ball.
- Preventive initiatives that focus on the sites of the body parts by sport are Cricket (Elbow, Shoulders, Fingers, Ankel, Thigh), Baseball (shoulder, ankle, hand, calf wrist), Kabaddi (knee, ankle, chin, elbow, fingers), Basketball (ankle, knee, elbow, shoulder), Hockey (knee, elbow, thigh, eyebrow, shin), Football (knee, ankle, thigh, calf, foot, elbow, shin and head), Wrestling (knee, elbow, fingers, ankle, ear and ribs), weight lifting (lumber vertebrae, palm, knee, thigh, shoulder), Badminton (knee, ankle, shoulder, elbow), Boxing (knuckles, nose, thumb, face, shoulder), Gymnastic (shoulder, hand, palm, knee, ankle), Judo (knee, face, ankle, shoulder, abdomen).
- Meniscus tear, ligament rupture, fracture, concussion and dislocation are most severe injuries found in various types of team and individual sports. Most of the injuries are minor, and moderate. Severe injuries are closely associated with highly stressful body contact and team sports such as, Boxing, Wrestling, Gymnastic, Basketball, Hockey, Football and Kabaddi.

- Percentages of match injuries are higher in team games and percentages of training injuries are higher in individual games.
- There is no significant difference found between new and recurrent injuries in team games and percentages of new injuries are higher in individual games.
- It is conclude that lack of knowledge towards sports injury and sport medicine may lead to recurrent injuries in various types of team and individual sports.
- Soft tissue injuries are most common and considered as minor injuries. The frequencies of soft tissue injuries are higher among all injuries in team and individual sports. Individual games have slightly higher frequencies in bone and joint injuries.
- Clay and grass courts are highly injury prone surfaces in various team and individual games and wooden surface was is considered as lowest injury prone surface.
- Improper warming-up, twist, fitness and jerk are most common intrinsic reasons in both team and individual sports.
- It is observed that most of the respondents do not know the exact reason of injuries occurred.
- Collision/Impact, fall or slip, field or playground, poor technique and unknown are the most frequent and common extrinsic reasons in various team and individual sports.
- The present study indicate that association between Abrasion, Incision, Laceration, Sprain, Strain and Concussion and game type are high. Except these injuries all other injuries and game type are independent mean there is no association between the occurrence of these injuries and game type.

V.4 RECOMMENDATIONS

This study conducted between team and individual sports competition. It is hoped that all the sports departments in India should come forward to adopt sports injury reporting system for documentation and for future research.

The resultant recommendations have been categorized as general prevention method of injuries in sports, and specific preventive methods.

V.4.1 General Methods of Preventions
The general recommendations have been classified as follow:

V.4.1.1 Physical Fitness
Good physical fitness is of the eventual important in dodging sports injuries. Whose basic physical fitness level is below normal are more prone to injuries. Regular exercise and general physical activities throughout the year can achieve a basic physical fitness level. General acclimatizing and training of large muscle groups is of great importance in most of the sports.

V.4.1.2 Warming-up and Cooling-down
The purposes behind warm up exercises are increase our range of motion of our joint and elasticity of our muscles which reduces the injury probability. Warm up increase muscle temperature, alertness and psychological preparation for the activity.

Cool down is also important as warming up which help a players in recover fast and washout the waste product after exercise.

V.4.1.3 Sports surfaces
It was observed that most common injury reason were impact, and fall or slip as we analyzed earlier in 4th chapter of this thesis. Quality sports surfaces reduce the slippery movement and improved cushioning especially landing from vertical movements. Most of the surfaces related to injuries were not well maintained.

V.4.1.4 Protective Equipment in Injury Prevention
A protective gear helps in reducing the chance of injury occurrence. But several factors affect the selection of protective gears. A protective gear is only effective when it meets the desired demands. It should be properly fitted. It should be made temperature absorbing material.

V.4.1.5 Knowledge of Rules

If a sportsperson follow the norms and standards made by the concerned authority he/she may certainly reduce the injury chance. It is only observation we have no any publication till now that knowledge of rules decrease the chance of injuries.

V.4.2 Specific injury prevalence methods

V.4.2.1 Injury Surveillance system

Information about the occurrences, nature of sports injuries and consciousness is the main product of injury surveillance. Injury surveillance is the first step in classifying the problem. Surveillance of injuries also helps in recognizing the cause of injuries so that injury prevention dealings can be developed as an intervention. This will permit for some injuries to be prevented. It is hoped that the coaches, administrators should appliance sports injury data collection system in their establishments that will help to develop injury prevention methodologies in all sports.

V.4.3 Curriculum Recommendation

New leanings in sports specific injury avoidance information be made accessible to referees, umpires, officials, coaches, Directors, teachers, players and parents about the nature and prevalence of sports injuries. Sports medicine should be a subjects in school or college students in their curriculum.

V.5 SUGGESTION FOR FURTHER RESEARCH

It is recommended that future researchers should focus on the following topics that bring appreciative between sports injuries and its avoidance, Supplementary researchers can go deep into the precise aspects of particular sport or situation.

[1] A study can be done on the different methods of strength training in prevention of sports injuries.

[2] A study can be done on therapeutic modalities in relation with particulars injuries.

[3] A similar study can be conducted on different sports.

[4] A similar study can be conducted on different sports and variables such as injury incidence rate, athlete exposures and clinical incidence etc.

[5] Strategies to reduce the incidence of head, neck, low back, spine injuries and necessary to design protective equipment.

[6] Psychological assessment of players after injury.

[7] Psychological factors affecting injuries in sports.

[8] Assessment of injuries in different games in relation to their playing position of team games.

[9] Duration of exposure in the play and its relationship to sports injuries in team Games.

[10] Relationship between sports facilities and injury occurrence.

BIBLIOGRAPHY

BIBLIOGRAPHY

Ajmer Singh, J. B. (2012). *ESSENTIAL OF PHYSICAL EDUCATION.* New Delhi: Kalyani Publishers.

Carol C. Teitz, M. (1989). *Scientific Foundations of Sports Medicine.* Washington: B.C. Decker Inc, South Service Road.

Colby, M. D. (2017). Preseason Workload Volume and High-Risk Periods for Noncontact Injury Across Multiple Australian Football League Seasons. *Journal of Strength and Conditioning Research, 31*(7), 1821-1829.

Dallinga, J., Benjaminse, A., & Lemmink, K. (2012). Which screening tools can predict injury to the lower extremities in team sports?: A systematic review. *Sports Medicine, 42*(9), 791-815.

Dictionary, Y. (2016). *Sports Medicine.* Retrieved from Your Dictionary : http://www.yourdictionary.com

Echlin, P. T. (2010). Return to play after an initial or recurrent concussion in a prospective study of physician-observed junior ice hockey concussions: implications for return to play after a concussion. *Neurosurgical focus, 29*(5), E5.

Gale, (2008). *Encyclopedia of Medicine.* Retrieved from Medical Dictionary: http://medical-dictionary.thefreedictionary.com

Garrick JG, R. R. (1978). *Injuries in High School Sports.Pediatrics.* Washington: Scientific Foundation of Sports Medicine.

Griffith, H. W. (1989). *Complete Guide to Sports Injuries.* New Delhi: Metropolitan Book Co. Pvt. Ltd.

Grinsogono, V. (1989). *INTERNATIONL PERPESPECTIVE IN PHYSICAL THERAPY.* NEW YORK: Churchill livingstone.

Harries, M. W. (1994). *OXFORD TEXT BOOK OF SPORTS MEDICINE.* New York: Oxford University Press.

Hootman, J., Dick, R., & Agel, J. (2007). Epidemiology of collegiate injuries for 15 sports: Summary and recommendations for injury prevention initiatives. *Journal of Athletic Training, 42*(2), 311-319.

Kalina, R., & Mosler, D. (2017). Risk of injuries caused by fall of people differing in age, sex, health and motor experience. *Advances in Intelligent Systems and Computing, 603,* 84-88.

Khanna, G. L., & Jayparkash, G. S. (1990). *Exercise Physiology and Sports Medicine.* Hisar: Lucky Enterprises.

Khatun, A. (2016). A study of selected sports injuries and their preventive and rehabilitative measures among women soccer players of west Bengal soccer clubs. *International Journal of Multidisciplinary Research and Development, 3*(1), 124-126.

Kovacic, J., & Bergfeld, J. (2005). Return to play issues in upper extremity injuries. *Clinical Journal of Sport Medicine, 15*(6), 448-452.

Kuzuhara, K., Shibata, M., & Uchida, R. (2016). Injuries in Japanese mini-basketball players during practices and games. *Journal of Athletic Training, 51*(12), 1022-1027.

Leung, F., & Smith, F. (2017). Injuries in Australian school-level rugby union. *Journal of Sports Sciences, 35*(21), 2088-2092.

Mayo foundation for Medical Education and Research (MFMER). (2017). *Diseases & Condition.* Retrieved May 20, 2017, from mayoclinic.org: www.mayoclinic.org

Mazer, B., Shrier, I., Feldman, D., Swaine, B., Majnemer, A., Kennedy, E., et al. (2010). Clinical management of musculoskeletal injuries in active Children and youth. *Clinical Journal of Sport Medicine, 20*(4), 249-255.

MedicineNet. (2017, 10 20). *Medical Definition of Fracture.* Retrieved 10 20, 2017, from medicinenet.com: https://www.medicinenet.com

Meurer, M., Silva, M., & Baroni, B. (2017). Strategies for injury prevention in Brazilian football: Perceptions of physiotherapists and practices of premier league teams. *Journal of Physical Therapy in Sport, 28,* 1-8.

Murray, I., Murray, S., Mackenzie, K., & Coleman, S. (2005). How evidence based is the management of two common sports injuries in a sports injury clinic? *British Journal of Sports Medicine, 39*(12), 912-916.

Orchard, J., & Hopkins, W. (2007). For debate: Consensus injury definitions in team sports should focus on missed playing time. *Clinical Journal of Sport Medicine, 17*(3), 192-196.

Pande, D. P. (1987). *OUTLINE OF SPORTS MEDICINE.* Gwalior: Jaypee Brothers, Medical Publishers.

Pandey, S. P. (2017). Prevention & management of specific sports injuries through Ayurveda. *International Journal of Yogic, Human Movement and Sports Sciences, 2*(1), 04-08.

Pastor, M., Ezechieli, M., Classen, L., Kieffer, O., & Miltner, O. (2015). Prospective study of injury in volleyball players: 6 year results. *Techology and Health Care, 23*(5), 637-643.

Pradeep T, S. S. (2016). The influence of dynamic stretch of quadriceps, hamstrings and its combined stretch effect on knee joint position sense (JPS) in healthy adults. *International Journal of Multidisciplinary Research and Development, 3*(10), 50-54.

Reynolds, B., & Patrie, J. (2017). Comparative analysis of head impact in contact and collision sports. *Journal of Neurotrauma, 34*(1), 38-49.

Schmikli, S. B. (2009). National survey on Sports Injuries in the Netherland: Target Populations for Sports Injury Prevention Programs. *Clinical Journal of Sports Medicine, 19*(2), 101-106.

Shaw, D., & Gambhir, S. (2000). *Encyclopaedia of Sports Injuries and Indian Sports Persons.* Delhi: Khel Sahitya Kendra.

Simbak, Q. G. (2017). Modified rehabilitation exercises to strengthen the gluteal muscles with a significant improvement in the lower back pain. *International Journal of Yoga, Physiotherapy and Physical Education, 2*(1), 20-24.

Spinks, A., & McClure, R. (2007). Quantifying the risk of sports injury: A systematic review of activity-specific rates for children under 16 years of age. *British Journal of Sports Medicine, 41*(9), 548-557.

Vijay. (2001). *Hand Book of Sports Medicine.* New Delhi: Friends Publications (India).

Vinger PF, H. E. (1986). *Sports Injuries-the Unthwarted Epidemic; 2nd ed.* Littleton, MA: PSG Publishing.

Wolpa, M. E. (1982). *The Sports Medicien Guide: treating and preventing common athletic injuries.* USA: Leisure Press.

Yang, C. L. (2016). Management of Sports Injuries with Korean Medicine: A Survey of Korean National Volleyball Team. *Evidence-Based complementary and Alternative Medicine.*

CPSIA information can be obtained
at www.ICGtesting.com
Printed in the USA
BVHW050923040123
655320BV00009BA/746